Clinical Practice and Economics

Contributors

Sir Douglas Black BSc DSc MD PRCP
Department of Health and Social Security, London

Professor J C Brocklehurst MD MSc FRCPEd FRCPGlas
Department of Geriatric Medicine, University of Manchester

Sir John Brotherston MA LLD MD DPH DrPH FRCPEd FRCPGlas FRSEd FFCM
Professor of Community Medicine, University of Edinburgh
Recently, Chief Medical Officer, Scotland

Wilfrid I Card MD FRCP FRCPEd FRCPGlas
Senior Research Fellow, University Department of Medicine, Western Infirmary, Glasgow
Late Professor, Department of Medicine in relation to Mathematics and Computing, University of Glasgow

Professor H A F Dudley ChM MB ChB FRCSEd FRACS
Surgical Unit, St Mary's Hospital, London

Fred Ederer BS MA
Chief, Office of Biometry and Epidemiology, National Eye Institute, Bethesda, Maryland, USA

Dr John Fry MD FRCS FRCGP
General Practitioner

Professor Bryan Jennett MD FRCS FRCSGlas FRSEd
Institute of Neurological Sciences, Southern General Hospital, Glasgow

Professor R E Kendell MD MRCP MRCPsych DPM
Institute of Psychiatry, Denmark Hill, London

Professor M G Kerr BSc MB ChB FRCOG FRCSEd
Department of Obstetrics and Gynaecology, University of Calgary, Alberta, Canada

W Morrice McCrae MB FRCPEd FRCPGlas
Consultant Physician, Royal Hospital for Sick Children, Edinburgh
Senior Lecturer, Department of Child Life and Health, University of Edinburgh

Professor E J Moran Campbell MD PhD FRCP FRCP(C)
Department of Medicine, McMaster University, Hamilton, Ontario, Canada

Dr I J T Parboosingh BSc MB ChB MRCOG
Department of Obstetrics and Gynaecology, University of Edinburgh

Professor L Mary Pickford MSc DSc MRCS LRCP FRSEd FRS
Professor Emeritus, University of Edinburgh
Special Professor of Endocrinology, University of Nottingham

W Duncan Reekie BCom PhD
Department of Business Studies, University of Edinburgh

Dr H R Rollin MD MRCP FRCPsych DPM
Department of Psychiatry, Horton Hospital, Epsom, Surrey

W T Thom OBE MB ChB DTM&H MFCM
Principal Medical Officer, Scottish Home and Health Department

Professor O L Wade MA MD FRCP FRCPI(Hon)
Department of Therapeutics and Clinical Pharmacology, University of Birmingham

Professor L G Whitby MA PhD MD FRCP FRCPEd FRCPath FRSEd
Department of Clinical Chemistry, University of Edinburgh

Professor Sir Michael Woodruff DSc MD MS FRCS FRS
Department of Surgery, University of Edinburgh

Clinical Practice and Economics

Edited by

C I Phillips MD, PhD, MSc, DPH, FRCS, FRCSEd
Professor of Ophthalmology
University of Edinburgh

and

J N Wolfe MA, BLitt
Professor of Economics
University of Edinburgh

PITMAN MEDICAL

First published 1977

Cat. No. 21 3008 81

Pitman Medical Publishing Co Ltd
42 Camden Road, Tunbridge Wells,
Kent, TN1 2QD, England

Associated Companies

UNITED KINGDOM
Pitman Publishing Ltd, London
Focal Press Ltd, London

USA
Fearon-Pitman Publishers Inc, California

AUSTRALIA
Pitman Medical Publishing Pty Ltd, Melbourne

CANADA
Pitman Publishing, Toronto
Copp Clark Publishing, Toronto

EAST AFRICA
Sir Isaac Pitman and Sons Ltd, Nairobi

NEW ZEALAND
Pitman Publishing NZ Ltd, Wellington

SOUTH AFRICA
Pitman Publishing Co SA (Pty) Ltd, Johannesburg

British Library Cataloguing in Publication Data
Clinical practice and economics.
1. Medical economics — Great Britain
I. Phillips, C I II. Wolfe, James Nathaniel
338.4'7'610941 RA410.55.G7

ISBN 0-272-79409-0

Set in 10/11 IBM Press Roman by Datalith Ltd, Edenbridge, Kent
and printed by offset litho and bound in
Great Britain at The Pitman Press, Bath, Avon

Contents

continued

Introduction

In less than 25 years (1951-1974) the cost of the National Health Service in Britain has nearly trebled, from £462 million in 1951 to £1298 million in 1974 (1), at 1950 prices. This is an increase in its share of the Gross National Product in the same period from 3.87 to 5.30 per cent.

There are many causes for the rising proportion of the Gross National Product which is absorbed by our National Health Service. New and more expensive techniques are constantly becoming available, the proportion and absolute numbers of the aged in the British population are increasing and the real income of staff of all kinds is rising.

It is one of our basic premises that greater economy and efficiency in the use of clinical resources is desirable and possible. We have invited clinicians in medical and surgical practice to discuss their specialties in their economic context. Many important clinical subjects are not represented for reasons of space. Non-clinical areas are also largely excluded, although more efficient organization and administration are clearly desirable. Health education and preventive medicine are almost completely ignored. However, we have included chapters on research, clinical chemistry, the randomized clinical trial and the epidemiology of geriatrics.

It is possible to argue that health should absorb more resources, especially with an increasing Gross National Product; nevertheless, we think that general and selective economies are still important in the clinical field. Our contributors should not be interpreted as advocating any general retreat in medicine but a reduction in the superfluous, ephemeral and ill-advised would provide greater opportunity to implement the advances which we confidently expect in the future.

We hope that our readers – doctors, students, nurses, administrators, economists and interested laymen – will find the chapters in this book interesting and stimulating.

Calbert I. Phillips
J.N. Wolfe

Reference

1. Office of Health Economics (1976). *Information Sheet* No. 29. July, Table 1.

Part One
Clinical Practice

1

The Randomized Clinical Trial

Fred Ederer

'If you are going to investigate the value of a treatment, how do you decide if it is any good or not?... If you do no more than say "what I say three times is true," i.e., if I say the patient has recovered he has recovered, and vice versa, then your reader has to decide whether he is interested in your opinion or not. If he is, he goes on reading, but if he is not, he turns over the page and that's that.'

M. Hamilton (1)

Opinion has always played an important role in the history of medicine, but today, more than ever before, there is a demand for scientific evidence on the value of therapeutic, prophylactic and diagnostic procedures in clinical medicine (2), and the scientific tool capable of producing this kind of evidence is the randomized controlled clinical trial (RCT). It came into prominence during the late 1940s, and Bradford Hill (now Sir Austin) is generally credited with introducing this technique. The President of the Royal College of Surgeons thought that this contribution of Hill's to medicine was as important and valuable as the discovery of penicillin (3).

The RCT is an application of statistical methods to medicine (4, 5). Its principles include reliance on objective findings rather than opinions or clinical impressions, study of disease in defined groups rather than in individuals, prevention of bias (by such devices as randomization and 'masking'), use of standardized rather than improvised diagnostic and therapeutic procedures, and formation of conclusions based on biometrically analyzed data rather than anecdotal information.

Medical training emphasizes the uniqueness of patients and the study of their distinctive characteristics. Users of statistical methods seek to describe quantitatively the common and variable elements of the disease, and how its development or course may be influenced by certain diagnostic, prophylactic or therapeutic interventions. Although the physician wants to know whether a certain type of intervention will help a *particular* patient, this question can usually not be answered because for many diseases patients tend to get better whether treated or not, and even in progressive diseases the course is often marked by spontaneous remissions. The RCT helps to establish not whether a certain form of medical intervention will or will not help a particular patient, but to what extent the intervention may influence, in *groups* of patients, the risk of disease, the likelihood of improvement, or the risk of complications and of end-points of the disease. As Runyon said, 'The race is not always to the swift, nor the battle to the strong – but that's the way to bet.'

Atkins (3) points out that it would be absurd not to admit that immense advances in therapeutic knowledge were made before 1945, 'but if we look at these critically we are bound to observe that the therapeutic measures which have stood the test of time, both medical and surgical, were discovered at infrequent intervals and were in what we might term the Nobel Prize class'. Atkins refers to such discoveries as lime juice for the treatment of scurvy, quinine for malaria, and penicillin, which led to results 'so striking and undeniable that no clinical trial was necessary to establish them firmly as therapeutic agents of the first magnitude'.

In contrast to these milestones in therapeutic medicine there were numerous treatments, introduced without proper evaluation, which at one time were widely practiced but later abandoned 'because they were ultimately found to be without value if not clearly harmful' (6). The list includes gastric freezing for peptic ulcer, colectomy for epilepsy, potassium arsenite for treatment of leukemia, bilateral hypogastric artery ligation for pelvic hemorrhage, mercury for the treatment of syphilis, portacaval shunt for hepatic cirrhosis, renal-capsule stripping for acute renal failure, sympathectomy for asthma, internal mammary artery ligation for coronary artery disease, the 'button' operation for ascites, adrenalectomy for essential hypertension, complete dental extraction for a variety of complaints thought to be the result of focal sepsis, and wiring for aortic aneurysm. According to the NIH Clinical Trials Committee (6), these treatments 'remained in medical practice too long, and frequently at very high cost in money and resources and to the detriment of patients'.

Methods of the RCT

Controls. The RCT is a scientific experiment. In the ideal experiment, the experimental and control units are identical except for the treatment, so that any difference in outcome must be attributable to the treatment. The first requirement of the RCT, then, is that, in addition to a treated series of patients, there be a *concurrent* control (comparison) series. Except for the rare 'Nobel Prize class' examples of dramatically effective treatments cited earlier, studies without controls are difficult and in many cases impossible to interpret. For example, in a trial of antihistamines, of colds under one day's duration, 13.4 per cent were cured and 68.2 per cent were cured or improved on the second day following antihistamine treatment; the corresponding control group (placebo) figures were 13.9 and 64.7 per cent (7). Could the antihistamine findings have been properly interpreted without controls? The control group may be seen as a yardstick without which the experimental procedure would have to be evaluated qualitatively, which the scientific method attempts to avoid.

Non-concurrent controls (i.e. historical controls) are suspect because conditions affecting the comparability of treated and control patients often change over time for known or unknown reasons. 'Diseases change in time, medical treatments change, and the indications for operations change' (8). Also, the sources of referred patients and the diagnostic acumen of referring physicians change. Despite some recent advocacy for historical controls under special circumstances (9), the prevailing opinion among scientists is that the RCT reigns supreme as a method of evaluating methods of clinical intervention (10). Concurrent controls prevent bias due to temporal factors.

Randomization. The second requirement of the RCT is that allocation of patients to concurrent treated and control groups be made at random. The objective is not to match individual patients, but rather to create groups which are on the whole similar. We may, without randomization, be able to match treated and control groups on characteristics which we know to be prognostically important. We cannot, however, match on prognostic factors which have not been identified as such or which we cannot observe or measure. Randomization tends to match on all factors, prognostic and non-prognostic, observable and non-observable, measurable and not measurable. Randomization, moreover, eliminates conscious and unconscious sources of bias in the selection of the group to be treated and, further, allows the use of statistical and probability theory in analyzing the results.

It should be stressed that alternate assignment of patients to one or the other treatment or assigning them to one treatment on odd days and to the other on even days are *not* methods of randomizing. Randomization means that the choice of treatment for each patient should be made by an independent act of randomization, such as the toss of a coin or the use of a table of random numbers. It is critical to the success of the RCT that the doctor not know what treatment is coming up, because if he knows, he has the chance to hedge on whether and when to admit the patient to the study. In a multiclinic trial of anticoagulant therapy using the odd/even calendar day method of assigning treatment, it was discovered that more patients than expected had been admitted on odd days; that treated cases were hospitalized earlier than control cases; and that a higher proportion of treated cases were private cases, had private duty nurses and were severe at onset. The method of assigning treatments thus failed to produce comparable groups, for which the most plausible explanation apparent to the investigators was that 'as physicians observed the benefits of anti-coagulant therapy, they speeded up, where feasible, the hospitalization of those patients ... who would routinely have been hospitalized on an even day in order to bring as many as possible under the odd-day deadline' (11).

Ethical Considerations. Is it ethical to randomize patients between a new therapy and the standard therapy? Chalmers (12) said that it is more ethical to randomize than to give 'a new or the standard therapy as if we knew that one or the other was better, when either might actually be more harmful than beneficial'. Davis (13) proposed that randomization is ethical when 'our best guess is that the chances of benefit and harm' of the new therapy are in balance. Still another criterion is that randomization is ethical when there is 'adequate collective doubt' about the relative value of a new therapy (14). It has become a standard requirement for patients who enter an RCT to sign a consent form which describes the nature and purpose of the study and the potential benefits and risks of the treatment.

Masking. The history of science abounds with examples of personal bias influencing the observations made both by the research subjects and by the investigators (15). Francis Bacon (16) summed it up in twelve words: 'For what a man had rather were true, he more readily believes.'

Investigators and patients have a stake in the outcome of a clinical trial, and this can influence their objectivity. Both patients and investigators may have a strong wish for the treatment to succeed; or, conversely, patients may enjoy secondary gains from failing to improve. 'Double-masking'* can prevent these psychological factors from influencing the outcome. In the double-masked study, neither the investigator nor the patient knows what treatment is being administered to an individual patient. When it is not feasible to mask the doctor, as for example when a treatment produces tell-tale side-effects, a 'single-masked' study, in which only the patient is masked, may nevertheless be feasible. The placebo is used as the double-masking device in medical trials, but in surgical trials it is not possible to mask the surgeon. When the treating physician cannot be masked, assessment of the outcome of treatment can still be unbiased if it is made by a masked examiner. In some surgical trials a sham procedure has been used to mask the patient.

Adequate Size of Study. The number of patients studied in a clinical trial should be large enough so that the results will be statistically meaningful. Requirements for the size of the study population should be determined in advance to prevent inconclusive findings (17). Often the number of

*'Double-blinding', an awkward term, is often used in lieu of 'double-masking'.

patients potentially available to a single clinic is too small, and it is then necessary to consider a multiclinic study. Multiclinic studies often involve, in addition to a number of clinical centers (one study, the Coronary Drug Project (18), involved 53 clinical centers), a co-ordinating center for central data collection and processing, a central laboratory or reading center (for such documents as electrocardiograms or x-rays), and an elaborate committee structure. The management complexities of multiclinic studies are formidable (19).

Well Defined Diagnostic and Therapeutic Procedures. In planning a clinical trial, it is important to define the criteria for patient eligibility so that one may be able to determine precisely to what class of patients the findings apply. For similar reasons, the methods of diagnosis, treatment and clinical assessment of the outcome of treatment must also be described in detail. If several studies of the same treatment of the disease result in conflicting findings, as often happens, it is important to be able to determine whether certain differences in criteria for selecting patients or certain differences in therapeutic or clinical assessment procedures could account for the discrepant findings. Within a study, the various clinical and laboratory procedures must be standardized, and the reproducibility of critical observations should be investigated. In multiclinic studies, centrally performed laboratory and photographic analyses can reduce observer error.

Biometric Methods of Data Analysis. The statistical analysis of the results should first consider whether the trial's various treatment groups are indeed comparable with respect to various prognostic factors. The possibility of lack of comparability, despite randomization and despite 'pre-stratification', cannot be ruled out, and if such dissimilarities exist, they should be dealt with in the data analysis with such statistical methods as 'post-stratification'.

The analysis should include a complete accounting of patients admitted to the study, i.e. a tabulation of drop-outs and other losses, such as deaths. Patients lost to follow-up may differ, in such prognostically important characteristics as age or severity of disease, from patients remaining under follow-up. Dorn (20) said, 'The validity of a follow-up study may be seriously impaired if every person is not observed for the maximum duration... Even a small percentage lost to follow-up ... may seriously bias the observations... The only correct way of handling persons lost to follow-up is not to have any.' The number and characteristics of patients lost to follow-up in the various treatment groups should be compared and the possible biasing influence of this incomplete information should be evaluated. The data analysis should also include an assessment of the statistical significance of the outcome.

Written Protocol. The plan of a clinical trial, including the nature and purpose of the study, the specific objectives, design and methods, is written down in great detail in a research protocol (21). The detail should be such that an independent investigator would be able to precisely replicate the study by merely following the written protocol.

Examples of the RCT

Clinical trials may be classified into therapeutic, prophylactic and diagnostic trials. The therapeutic trial evaluates treatments of disease; the prophylactic trial evaluates preventive measures, such as vaccines; and the diagnostic trial evaluates the efficacy of diagnostic procedures, such as mammography. When well done, these trials can answer timely questions and advance our understanding of the disease, its treatment or its prevention – whether the findings are positive or negative. And both positive and negative findings can lead to either an increase or a decrease in the costs of medical care (22). Some examples, first of negative and then of positive findings, will illustrate these concepts.

In a recent carefully conducted double-masked trial, patients with severe viral hepatitis were randomly assigned to corticosteroid (methylprednisolone) or placebo therapy (23). Seven of the 14 patients assigned to corticosteroid and 2 of the 15 assigned to placebo died during the 16-week study period. With the excess mortality in the steroid-treated patients not reaching conventional levels of statistical significance (p=.08), the investigators cautiously concluded that 'methylprednisolone does not enhance survival in patients with severe viral hepatitis, and it may be detrimental'. They also point out that while corticosteroid therapy has been widely used in treating viral hepatitis since 1951, its efficacy has never been demonstrated in a clinical trial, and they recommend discontinuing this treatment 'until further studies confirm or deny' their results.

Gastric 'freezing' for treating duodenal ulcer, requiring a costly, expensive to operate hypothermia machine, was introduced in 1962. Initial enthusiasm for this treatment was followed by scepticism, and in 1969 the results of a randomized, double-masked study of 160 patients showed the 'freezing' procedure to be no better than a sham procedure with respect to relief of pain, secretory suppression, number and severity of recurrences, or development of certain defined deleterious outcomes ('end-points') (24). The investigators concluded that the psychologic effect of the procedure probably explained the findings of relief of pain and subjective improvement in earlier studies.

The Coronary Drug Project, a randomized, double-masked trial involving more than 8,000 American men tested the hypothesis that reducing blood cholesterol after recovery from a heart attack can prolong life. Of the five drugs studied, three were discontinued early because they appeared to cause more harm than good. The two remaining drugs – niacin and clofibrate – although they lowered blood cholesterol, failed to influence mortality significantly. After an average follow-up of more than 6 years, the death rates were 25.5, 24.4 and 25.4, respectively, in the clofibrate, niacin and placebo groups (18). Despite the negative findings, the highest American health official has held that 'the outcome has significant implications for individuals who have survived a heart attack and are still receiving such therapy under the assumption of a favorable benefit/risk ratio. If this carefully controlled clinical trial had not been conducted, it is likely that the hazardous side effects of the therapy would still be attributed to the natural course of the disease rather than to the drugs themselves. In this instance, a clinical trial also pointed the way to a reduction in health care costs by as much as $200 to $300 million annually' (22).

Now a few examples of studies with positive findings. Photocoagulation treatment for proliferative diabetic retinopathy, a major cause of blindness, was introduced in 1959. During the next 15 years the treatment became widely accepted without adequate evidence of its value to the patient. Although numerous studies were published, none incorporated randomization or acknowledged the implementation of masking procedures, and only four used concurrent controls and drew conclusions about the effect of the treatment on visual acuity. Of these, two found some benefit of the treatment and two found no effect (25). In 1972 a multiclinic research group started a randomized trial of more than 1,700 patients with efforts to 'mask' the visual acuity examiner. The first results of that study showed the 2-year risk of blindness to be 16.3 per cent in untreated eyes and 6.4 per cent in treated eyes (26). How medical care costs will be affected by these findings is not yet known, but it is safe to assume that they will not decrease. The number of persons in the USA who face possible loss of vision from diabetic retinopathy was estimated to be more than 300,000 (27), and the cost of photocoagulation treatment is about $500-$1,500.

An example of a prophylactic trial is the 1954 United States field trial of the Salk poliomyelitis vaccine, 'the biggest public health experiment ever' (28). The incidence rate of poliomyelitis was found to be 50 per cent lower in some 200,000 school children who had been randomly selected for vaccination than in a corresponding group of placebo controls.

The final example is a diagnostic trial. In 1963 a long-term randomized trial was started to determine whether periodic breast cancer screening with mammography and clinical examination can reduce mortality from breast cancer in women. Some 62,000 women aged 40 to 64 years were randomized to either a study or a control group. Study group women were offered an initial screening examination and three additional annual screening examinations, while women in the control group followed their usual medical care practices. The investigation employed procedures designed to yield similar degrees of reliability in the identification of breast cancer cases and deaths among women in the two groups. After 7 years, breast cancer mortality under age 50 was about the same in the two groups but at age 50 or more it was some 40 per cent lower in the study group (Table 1.1) (29). Mammographic screening for breast

Table 1.1.
Breast cancer deaths by age at death, 7 years from date of entry

Age at death	*Control*	*Study*
40-49	16	17
50-59	59	32
60+	33	21

cancer is now generally recommended in the USA for women aged 50 or more and also in younger women who may be at high risk for breast cancer. There is disagreement on how the presence of certain high risk characteristics should be balanced against the possible hazards of low-dose radiation of the asymptomatic young woman.

Randomized clinical trials are immensely difficult (19) and the costs and resources required are 'staggering' (22). But Frederickson (14) called them the 'indispensable ordeal';

> 'They lack glamor; they strain our resources and patience, and they protract to excruciating limits the moment of truth. Still, they are among the most challenging tests of our skills. I have no doubt that when the problem is well chosen, the study is appropriately designed, and all the populations concerned made aware of the route and the goal, the reward can be commensurate with the effort. If, in major medical dilemmas, the alternative is to pay the cost of perpetual uncertainty, have we really any choice?'

References

1. Hamilton, M. (1961). *Methodology of Clinical Research.* Edinburgh and London, Churchill Livingstone.
2. Cochrane, A.L. (1972). *Effectiveness and Efficiency.* London, Nuffield Provincial Hospitals Trust.
3. Atkins, H. (1966). Conduct of a controlled clinical trial. *British Medical Journal,* **2,** 377-379.
4. Hill, A.B. (1962). *Statistical Methods in Clinical and Preventive Medicine.* Edinburgh and London, Churchill Livingstone.
5. Ederer, F. (Editor) (1975). The randomized controlled clinical trial. National Eye Institute Workshop for Ophthalmologists. *American Journal of Ophthalmologists,* 79, 752-789.
6. NIH Clinical Trials Committee (1976). Clinical Trial and the Public's Interest. Unpublished document. Jan. 23.
7. Special Committee of the Medical Research Council (1950). Clinical trials of antihistaminic drugs in the prevention and treatment of the common cold. *British Medical Journal,* **2,** 425.

8. Ballintine, E.J. (1975). Objective measurements and the double-masked procedure. *American Journal of Ophthalmology,* 79, 763-767.
9. Gehan, E.A. and Freireich, E.J. (1974). Non-randomized controls in cancer clinical trials. *New England Journal of Medicine,* 290, 198-203.
10. Byar, D.P., Simon, R.M., Friedewald, W.T., Schlesselman, J.J., DeMets, D.L., Ellenberg, J.H., Gail, M.H. and Ware, J.H. (1976). Randomized clinical trials. Perspectives on some recent ideas. *New England Journal of Medicine,* 295, 74-80.
11. Wright, I.S., Marple, C.D. and Beck, D.F. (1954). *Myocardial Infarction. Its Clinical Manifestations and Treatment with Anticoagulants,* pp. 9-11. New York, Grune and Stratton.
12. Chalmers, T.C. (1975). Ethical aspects of clinical trials. *American Journal of Ophthalmology,* 79, 753-758.
13. Davis, M.D. (1975). Applications of the principles of clinical trials. *American Journal of Ophthalmology,* 79, 779-785.
14. Frederickson, D.S. (1968). The field trial: some thoughts on the indispensable ordeal. *Bulletin of the New York Academy of Medicine,* 44, 985-993.
15. Ederer, F. (1975). Patient bias, investigator bias and the double-masked procedure. *American Journal of Medicine,* 58, 295-299.
16. Bacon, F. 'Aphorisms.' *Novum Organum.*
17. Halperin, M., Rogot, E., Gurian, J. and Ederer, F. (1968). Sample sizes for medical trials with special reference to long-term therapy. *Journal of Chronic Diseases,* 21, 13-24.
18. Coronary Drug Research Group (1975). Clofibrate and niacin in coronary heart disease. *Journal of the American Medical Association,* 231, 360-381.
19. Ederer, F. (1975). Practical problems in collaborative clinical trials. *American Journal of Epidemiology,* 102, 111-118.
20. Dorn, H.F. (1950). Methods of analysis for follow-up studies. *Human Biology,* 22, 238-248.
21. Bearman, J.E. (1975). Writing the protocol for a clinical trial. *American Journal of Ophthalmology,* 79, 775-778.
22. Cooper, T. (1976). Clinical trials – bridging basic research and applied health care. *American Society for Microbiology News,* 42, 662-663.
23. Gregory, P.B., Knauer, M., Kempson, R.L. and Miller, R. (1976). Steroid therapy in severe viral hepatitis. *New England Journal of Medicine,* 294, 68-687.
24. Ruffin, J.M., Grizzle, J.E., Hightower, N.C., McHardy, G., Shull, H. and Kirsner, J.B. (1969). A co-operative double-blind evaluation of gastric 'freezing' in the treatment of duodenal ulcer. *New England Journal of Medicine,* 281, 16-19.
25. Ederer, F. and Hiller, R. (1975). Clinical trials, diabetic retinopathy, and photocoagulation. A reanalysis of five studies. *Survey of Ophthalmology,* 19, 267-286.
26. Diabetic Retinopathy Study Research Group (1976). Preliminary report on effects of photocoagulation therapy. *American Journal of Ophthalmology,* 81, 1-14.
27. Morris, J.M. (1975). Unpublished document. National Eye Institute, Bethesda, Md, USA.
28. Meier, P. (1972). The biggest public health experiment ever: the 1954 field trial of the Salk poliomyelitis vaccine. In: *Statistics: A Guide to the Unknown.* Ed. by J.M. Tanur and others. San Francisco, Holden-Day.
29. Shapiro, S. (1974). Cohort studies: In populations covered by a comprehensive medical care system. *Excerpta Medica International Congress Series,* No. 351, Vol. 3, Florence.

2

Primary and Continuing Care

John Fry

Common Dilemmas and Common Goals

Blind euphoria in the prevention, control and management of disease is unrealistic. The World Health Organization's definition of 'health' as 'a state of physical, mental and social well-being and not merely an absence of disease' is a blissful Utopian target as is 'medical care as a human right and expectation'. We must all agree with these as desirable principles and objectives, but if we are to avoid frustration and anger of the public, the politicians and the medical profession, then we must be honest and admit that such common goals are non-achievable at present. We all are faced with common problems and common dilemmas.

There is within medical care an *insoluble equation.* It is not possible to match or equate public and professional 'wants' with political or professional estimates of 'needs' and even these with current available 'resources'. The provision of medical care soon becomes a bottomless pit of public or private costs unless some firm, but benevolent, controls are established and priorities agreed upon from reliable studies, experiments and collection of data.

Our common goals must be to endeavour to provide maximal care at minimal cost in balance with available resources and in keeping with a non-extravagant definition of our true needs of medical care.

Our common approach and endeavours must be to arrive at degrees of priorities that are acceptable to both the public and the profession, and within these to provide facilities for essential needs but at the same time to restrict care and services for non-essentials and to avoid the use of non-proven methods and techniques.

A common challenge to the profession is to adopt and apply in every-day normal practice modern critical and scientific methods through which only useful and proven methods of care are employed, and wasteful and placebo measures avoided.

Levels of Care

Within every health care system there are, and there have to be, four essential levels of care. There is personal and family *self-care.* At least three symptoms out of four are self-managed, and one-third of all expenditure on drugs in developed societies is for self-prescribed over-the-counter medication.

Then there is the first level of professional care, *primary care.* In Britain in the National Health Service this is provided by general practitioners, but in other health systems this primary care may be given by various specialists or 'specialoids', by nurses, by medical assistants or by other indigenous paramedical workers. Good primary care acts to protect the more specialized hospital services from inappropriate work, and serves also to protect the patients from unnecessary hazards at the hands of inappropriate specialist and hospital care.

General specialist care is based on a district hospital. The population of the district, around 250,000, has to be large enough to warrant the services of general surgeons, general physicians (internists), paediatricians, obstetricians, gynaecologists, psychiatrists and supporting radiologists, pathologists and anaesthetists.

Super- (or sub-) specialist care for more rare diseases or problems requires a regional population of 1 - 5 million for units to deal with, for example, thoracic disorders, neurological and neurosurgical problems, plastic surgery.

Primary Care

There are certain special features of primary care (general practice). All systems and the roles and objectives must be related to these features.

The general practitioner (primary health worker) provides direct access to his patients at all times, or he makes arrangements for a deputy. He is involved in first contact that requires primary diagnosis and assessment of the whole patient in the context of his family and community environment before proceeding to treatment. The population for which the general practitioner is responsible is small, an average of 2,500 persons in the NHS, and relatively static. Only 10 per cent move in any year in the UK. Therefore, the general practitioner is able to provide long-term and continuing care over two or three generations and he gets to know his patients and the families well.

The nature and content of the work of general practice is that which occurs in a population of 2,500 at any time. Therefore, it is inevitable that the emphasis will be more on the common minor and chronic disorders and less on the more rare acute major and dramatic diseases.

Table 2.1 shows what a general practitioner in the British NHS can expect to see in his practice of 2,500 persons in a year. Such a pattern is different in emphasis from hospital experience.

Table 2.1
Expected annual morbidity in a typical general practice in the British NHS

Diseases	*Persons consulting per year in a population of 2500*
Minor diseases	
Upper respiratory infections	600
Anxiety, depression, personality problems	250
Skin infections, eczema, warts and urticaria	200
Acute diarrhoea/vomiting, dyspepsias, constipation	150
Chronic illnesses	
Chronic rheumatism	100
High blood pressure	50
Obesity	40
Chronic bronchitis	35
Migraine	30
Asthma	25
Peptic ulcers	20
Epilepsy	10
Diabetes	10
Thyroid disease	7
Parkinsonism	3
Multiple sclerosis	2
Chronic renal failure	<1
Acute major illnesses	
Acute bronchitis and pneumonia	80
Myocardial infarction	8
Appendicitis	5
Cancers (new)	5
Strokes (new)	5

One of the keystones of good care in any clinical field is a sound knowledge of the nature, course and outcome of the conditions that the doctor is treating. He must know the natural history of the common diseases. Only in this way can he decide what is curable, what is treatable, what is preventable and what is normal. From his personal knowledge of his patients he will know what is tolerable for them.

Much unnecessary care and expense is undertaken in the forlorn hope and impossible attempt to treat many conditions that are 'non-curable'. More honesty and less therapeutic endeavours would be of benefit not only to the patient's comfort but also to his pocket and to the national exchequer.

There are some diseases which improve spontaneously. There are some which are an inevitable part of the ageing process. There are some which, once present, go through a predictable period of activity and then regress naturally, and there are some which remain unchanged whatever the treatment. I have been able to define these patterns of natural history over 25 years of observations in my practice (1, 2, 3, 4).

Work in General Practice

One of the special opportunities in the British NHS is that it is possible to measure the number of consultations and home visits in general practice for a known registered population. This gives a measure of work that can be compared between various practices and areas.

Work in general practice so measured is variable and dynamic. The Royal College of General Practitioners (5) and the Office of Population Censuses and Surveys (6) have reported on annual consultation rates involving many general practices throughout the United Kingdom. There is a range from almost six consultations and home visits per person per year in some practices to less than two such consultations in others. There are many local factors that influence such rates, such as morbidity and social influences, age structure, and environmental and geographical characteristics. However, when allowances are made for such obvious regional factors there are still differences between general practices – in the same areas and even in the same localities.

Further analyses suggest that important factors that control the volume of work carried out by individual general practitioners are influenced by their own patterns of organization, philosophies and methods and techniques of work. Thus, for given comparable index diseases and situations, one practitioner may see the patient once and another three or four times, both with the same satisfactory outcome. Obviously it is of considerable economic importance to determine whether the high work rates of some practices can be reduced and whether the low rates of others are compatible with good care.

In my own practice, records over the past 25 years (Fig. 2.1) show that the work per patient has been halved and now I am able to look after twice as many patients in the same amount of time as in the past. My standards do not appear to have changed as far as the outcome of care is involved. The greatest fall has been in the reduction of home visits, by tenfold, but there was also a reduction of office consultations by one-third. The reasons for this dramatic reduction have been better organization, more delegation to paramedical colleagues, a better understanding of the natural history of the diseases that I was treating and more involvement of the patient in his or her own care.

Similar trends in the reduction of work in general practice have been reported by the Royal College of General Practitioners (5), where records from 12 practices over 10 years or more show an overall reduction of work load of 27 per cent – 60 per cent in home visits and 16 per cent in office consultations. The work in general practice as recorded in two national surveys by the General Register Office (7) and the Office of Population Censuses and Surveys (6) showed a fall of 25 per cent.

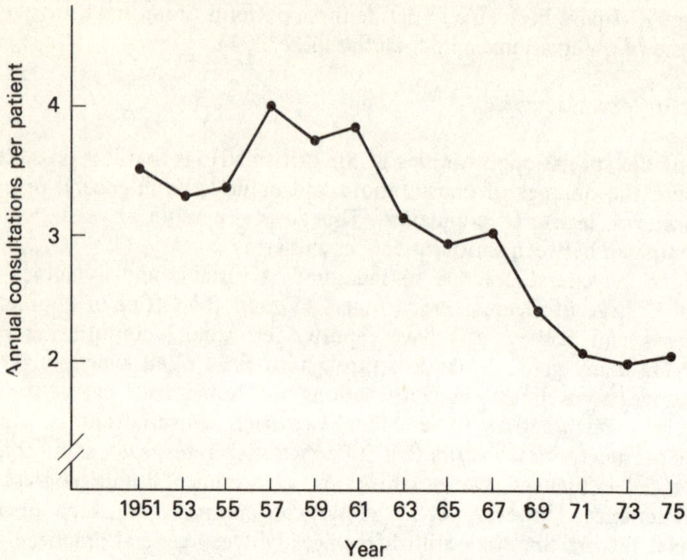

Figure 2.1 Volume of work in a general practice, 1950–1975

Self-care

We know that in 1974 £150 million was spent by the public on self-medication and a further £312 million on drugs prescribed by general practitioners in the NHS. In the USA the respective amounts spent were £2 billion and £5 billion (8).

Self-care is a field worthy of more study and research because it is possible that the more effective that self-care is the more healthy will be the public and the less expensive the health service.

Medical Manpower Needs

I have estimated that the life-career capital costs of a physician add up to £1 million (9). It is therefore an expensive step to admit a student into a medical school where the undergraduate training now costs £20,000. The numbers of medical students in Britain and in many other countries have been increased considerably in the belief that there is a great shortage of doctors. In Britain the numbers of new medical students entering medical schools are to increase from 2,289 in 1973 to 4,100 by 1980. This increase will add nearly £2,000 million expenditure to the national budget over the next half century.

I do not believe that there is enough evidence to show that we need this great increase in numbers of doctors. There are probably now more than enough general practitioners in the NHS. This is all the more valid in view of the falling work-load in general practice already noted.

The manpower situation in hospital practice is fraught with unknowns and uncertainties. Since no reliable work-studies have been carried out in hospitals we do not know the true number of senior, less senior and junior hospital staff required.

What we do know now is that with a population that is not increasing we need annually 1,815 new doctors to replace deaths and retirements from the NHS. If we add to this emigration, less than full-time work by the 30-40 per cent of women who are now entering our medical schools and to allow a growth of 2-3 per cent, then we will need 2,580 medical students graduating each year. This is far less than the 4,100 proposed. In my opinion there is a serious danger of medical unemployment or underemployment in 10 or 20 years' time.

Prescribing

In 1974 £272 million worth of drugs were prescribed by 21,000 general practitioners in England (10). This means that each general practitioner was responsible for £12,500 of drugs for his 2,500 patients or £5 per patient. This is much more than his gross income. The national drug bill is increasing by 5 per cent each year.

What are these drugs that are being prescribed at this tremendous rate? On average each person in Britain received five to six prescriptions each year at a cost of just under £1 per prescription. A very high proportion, almost half, must be given without the patient being seen, as a 'repeat' or 'unseen' prescription, because the average annual consultation rate is three to four per year.

Table 2.2 shows the number of prescriptions issued by general practitioners in 1974 in England and their total costs. It is justifiable to ask whether, in a population of 46.5 million, there really is need for 17 million prescriptions for hypnotics, 20 million for tranquillizers, 38 million for antibiotics, 7 million for laxatives and 5 million for vitamins.

There is an urgent need to review the enormous growth of general practice prescribing. The number of prescriptions per person has increased by 20 per cent in the past 15 years and the costs by 450 per cent. Surely there are strong indications for investigations, controlled trials and general questioning on whether all the prescriptions issued really are necessary, or beneficial?

However, the difficulties and dilemmas facing the general practitioners must be appreciated also because he is faced with patient demands and expectations that he cannot satisfy without a prescription.

It is salutary also to know that in spite of these high rates and costs they are lower than similar rates in other developed countries.

Table 2.2
Numbers and costs of prescriptions issued by general practitioners in 1974 in England (population 46.5 million)
Source: Annual Report from DHSS (HMSO)

Therapeutic group	*Number of prescriptions (in millions)*		*Total net ingredient costs (in millions)*	
Alimentary system		20		11
Laxatives	7		4	
Cardiovascular system		30		39
Diuretics	11		11	
Antihypertensives	6		11	
Lower respiratory system		27		20
Expectorants	17		5	
Antispasmodics	8		7	
Nervous system		74		40
Analgesics	19		10	
Hypnotics	17		6	
Tranquillizers	20		8	
Antidepressants	8		7	
Antibiotics		38		30
Nutrition and blood		14		7
Vitamins	5		2	
Skin		18		11
Corticosteroids	10		7	
Totals		274		205 (Total cost of prescriptions £275)

Reproduced by permission of the Controller of HMSO (10).

Medication – How Necessary?

As a personal contribution to the question of the non-necessity of much of the current medication by the medical profession, I make the following comments based on observations and studies in my own practice.

I believe that only about one-half of all *hypertensives* require specific treatment with antihypertensives in a carefully selected manner (3, 4, 11).

Angina is a relatively benign condition in general practice (12) and many patients so affected improve spontaneously over the years. The results of treating selected patients with *acute myocardial infarction* at home are as good as those treated in hospital (2).

The *'acute back'* will settle with rest, and masterly inactivity by the physician, within a few weeks in three cases out of four (13).

In general practice, *acute urinary infections* in women are frequent and benign. Many settle without specific therapy, some require chemotherapy and almost none leads to chronic renal infection or failure.

A law of three-thirds applies to the *common emotional disorders* in general practice. One-third suffer one attack and have no further troubles, one-third suffer occasional repeated episodes and one-third are chronic and do not respond well to any form of treatment from whatever source.

These are examples of how a knowledge of the natural history of diseases helps in more selective therapeutic approaches.

Referrals to Hospitals

The hospital service is the most expensive part of any health system. It is the general practitioners who control the use of the hospitals through their referrals. The numbers have tended to increase annually. In 1974, 11 per cent of all persons in Britain were admitted to a hospital, 17 per cent attended a specialist out-patient clinic as a new patient and 18 per cent attended at a hospital accident and emergency department. In the past four years the rates have levelled off.

These rates should be reducible. In my own practice my referrals to hospital specialists have been reduced by more than half over 25 years (Fig. 2.2).

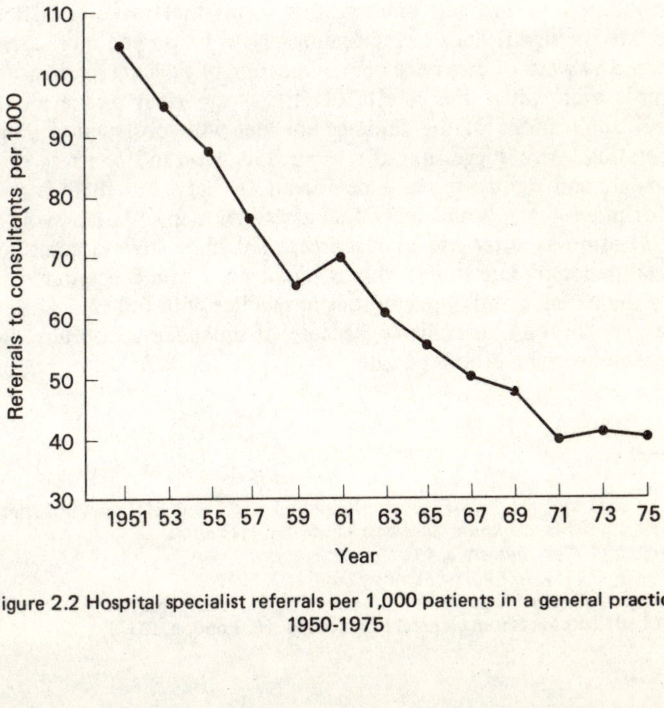

Figure 2.2 Hospital specialist referrals per 1,000 patients in a general practice, 1950-1975

The reasons are difficult to define but they must relate to an increasing confidence and experience of a general practitioner working in one practice over many years.

Discussion

In striving to create and to maintain good medical care for the communities in which we serve, a balance has to be achieved between professional idealism and economic realities. The 'art of the possible' applies with even more force to the provision of health care than to the realm of politics.

An examination of the present state of health economics reveals a number of major deficiencies. First, there is the abysmal lack of reliable and relevant data on which to base decisions for planning and action. Even in a National Health Service, such as the British model, after almost 30 years, there are gross deficiencies of information and intelligence on vital subjects such as use and deployment of medical manpower, on the use and effectiveness of current habits and methods of prevention and treatment and on an understanding of the nature and natural history of common disorders, to serve as a baseline by which to assess the need for and the success of medical care.

Second, there is a lack of understanding of the implications of the data that are available and there is a mass of this in official places. There is the general defect of unintelligible data. Reports of studies are presented and published in dull and uninteresting forms that make it difficult to appreciate the significance of the findings. New, better and more attractive and practical ways of in-service communication of data are necessary.

Third, even when the results of studies are clear and evident, the medical applications of the findings are met with obstruction and non-co-operation. Any suggestion for more directives and controls must be unpopular, and rightly so, in a democratic society, but there is a strong case for more controls and individual assessments in order to avoid waste and to promote better use of resources. This may involve some loss of 'clinical freedom' but unless this is based on a sound economic health service there may be no opportunities to practice with full clinical freedom if resources become unavailable because of squanderings on uneconomic medical and social methods of care.

References

1. Fry, J. (1966) *Profiles of Disease*. Edinburgh and London, Churchill Livingstone.
2. Fry, J. (1974). *Common Diseases*. Lancaster, MTP Press.
3. Fry, J. (1974). *Lancet*, 2, 431.
4. Fry, J. (1975). *Journal of Family Practice*, 2, 327.
5. Royal College of General Practitioners (1973). *Present State and Future Needs*, 3rd edn., Report from General Practice No. 16. London, RCGP.

6. Office of Population Censuses and Surveys (1974). *Second Morbidity Survey, 1970-71.* London, HMSO.
7. Logan, W.P.D. and Cushion, A.A. (1958). *Morbidity Statistics from General Practice.* London, HMSO.
8. Silverman, M. and Lee, P.R. (1974). *Pills, Profits and Politics.* Berkeley, University of California Press.
9. Fry, J. (1975). *Update,* **11**, 263.
10. DHSS (1976). *Health and Personal Social Services Statistics for England 1975.* London, HMSO.
11. Fry, J. (1975). *Journal of the Royal College of General Practitioners,* **25**, 481.
12. Fry, J. (1976). *Journal of the Royal College of General Practitioners,* **26**, 643-646.
13. Dillane, J.B., Fry, J. and Kalton, G. (1966). *British Medical Journal,* **2**, 82.

3

Effects of Intervention in Obstetrics

M.G. Kerr and I.J.T. Parboosingh

Four mothers and 60 babies died for every 1,000 births registered in England and Wales in 1928; during the next 20 years mortality rates associated with childbirth remained alarmingly high although there was some improvement during the war years. It is, therefore, understandable that a reduction in the number of deaths became the major objective of the obstetric service during the first 20 years of the National Health Service. The maternal and perinatal mortality rates have fallen steadily since 1946, while the State has invested an ever increasing proportion of its gross national product in the Maternity Services. The control of sepsis by antibiotics, the development of blood transfusion services, and improved anaesthesia, all contributed to the initial fall in maternal mortality, but in more recent years changes in the age, parity and general health of the parturient population have played a more important role. The falling perinatal mortality rate during this period has also been attributed to improved obstetric services, although direct evidence in support of this claim does not exist. However, encouraged by this common but unsubstantiated assumption, several official committees have advised the government to pursue a policy promoting hospital confinements and an increasing use of the specialist obstetric services. As a consequence, more than 80 per cent of all deliveries in the UK now take place in specialist hospitals and most prenatal care, especially in late pregnancy, is carried out by specialist obstetricians, while the community midwifery service and the general practitioner have played a steadily diminishing secondary role.

This pattern of care has evolved on the assumption that improvements in the staffing and organization of specialist hospitals have been mainly responsible for the fall in perinatal mortality and morbidity, although there is little evidence in support of a causal association. The work of Sir Dugald Baird and his colleagues in Aberdeen (1) and the results of the National Perinatal Mortality Surveys of 1946, 1958 and 1970 (2, 3) strongly suggest that the causes of perinatal mortality can be regarded as falling into two broad groups: those due to the effect of unfavourable environmental influences on the reproductive capacity of the mother (the environmental group), over which doctors have no direct control; and those associated with the type of complications of pregnancy and labour which can be prevented by competent obstetric skill (the obstetric group). Baird concluded that the significantly higher perinatal death rates in the north of Britain compared to the south were attributable to excessive death rates due to environmental rather than obstetric causes. The low perinatal death rates in Holland have also been attributed to the superior height and good health and the lower incidence of CNS malformations in Dutch women compared with British women. In summary, the evidence suggests that while the specialist obstetric services have played a substantial role in reducing maternal mortality and morbidity over the past 40 years, their contribution to the reduction in perinatal mortality which has taken place over this period is not so clearly defined and changes in the socioeconomic status and general health of the parturient population may have made the greater contribution.

The effect of obstetric intervention on perinatal morbidity is less clearly understood. Perhaps the most significant change in clinical obstetric practice in the UK in the past 15 years has been a dramatic increase in the incidence of induction of labour. In England and Wales the incidence increased from 15.8 per cent in 1964 to 33.5 per cent in 1972 (4) and many hospitals have since recorded induction rates greater than 50 per cent. The results of a controlled trial in Glasgow (5) on routine induction of labour at term suggested that this policy led to a significant reduction in the stillbirth rate in post-term pregnancies. However, Chalmers, Ziosnikje and Campbell (6) reached a different conclusion after analysing the outcome of nearly 40,000 deliveries to women in the Cardiff area over the period 1966-1972. During this period the induction rate increased by a factor of three but the perinatal mortality rate remained unchanged. It may be that the different results reflect differences in the populations in these two regions. It can also be remarked that the results of the Cardiff study suggest that antepartum monitoring of the fetus by oestrogen assays and serial ultrasound cephalometry made little impression on the outcome of pregnancy, although it would be unfortunate if these relatively new innovations were to be condemned before adequately controlled trials have been completed.

The effect of obstetric intervention on infant morbidity rates has been the subject of much debate. It is frequently argued that intensive prenatal and intrapartum care will reduce the incidence of mental and physical handicap in the community. On the other hand, the findings of the Peel Committee (7) could be held to suggest that a reduction in perinatal mortality due to intensive obstetric care might only lead to an increase in the incidence of handicapped children, as infants who would previously have died in utero or during the neonatal period would now survive. In fact, there is no evidence in support of either hypothesis. The prevalence of handicap has remained very constant over several decades. Abramowics and Richardson (8) reviewed 27 community studies between 1929 and 1969 and showed a prevalence rate of 4 per 1,000 children, which had remained constant over this period in spite of changes in obstetric practice. This is consistent with the findings of Fairweather and Illsley (9), who studied the birth histories of a group of subnormal children born in Aberdeen during a single year and concluded that the direct contribution of obstetric complications to the total volume of mental handicap is small. These workers emphasized that prematurity and low birth weight associated with placental malfunction were as important as birth injury in contributing to perinatal mortality and morbidity.

Several methods of monitoring of fetal well-being during pregnancy have become accepted as a routine part of clinical practice before they have been validated either by randomized controlled trials or equivalent procedures. Most studies to date have been on hospital-based populations and there have been difficulties in controlling the many variables which influence the final outcome. Many factors other than obstetric care improve the outcome of pregnancy by improving the quality of the parturient population – family planning, sterilization and abortion rates amongst low socioeconomic groups, changes in the fetal deformity rate as a result of prenatal screening, improved paediatric services, and changes in the social characteristics of the populations surrounding individual hospitals. Without advocating a retreat back to medieval practices, it remains to be established that sophisticated methods of assessment of fetal welfare have influenced pregnancy outcome.

There are many areas within the maternity services which are amenable to cost-benefit analysis and it is most unfortunate that this method of evaluation has been used only rarely by Health Service planners (10). For example, the costs and economic benefits of screening for and the termination of pregnancies with Down's syndrome and spina bifida cystica in women in the west of Scotland have been estimated (11, 12). The results of this study confirm the clinical impression that the greater the potential risk, the greater the economic benefits likely to accrue from prenatal screening. Hence, the potential economic benefits would be greater than the costs of screening for Down's syndrome in women aged 40 and over, probably equal to costs for those aged 35 and over, but less than the costs if the service were extended to women under the age of 35. It is important to appreciate that these estimates are based on the assumption that the organization of prenatal care ensures that all women are offered the test and wish to accept the offer. However, recent information suggests that less than half of the mothers over 40 years of age in the west of Scotland were in fact tested. The interpretation and application of cost-benefit analysis per se is, therefore, of limited value until more adequate promotion of good prenatal care is launched to ensure that pregnancy is diagnosed sufficiently early for the test to be carried out, and that doctors and midwives are aware that the tests are available; the explanation of the test to the patient must also be adequate to ensure that the majority of patients who would wish the affected pregnancy terminated accept the offer of amniocentesis. These comments lead to our belief that any form of intervention in the prenatal period will make greater economic sense if it is administered within a comprehensive perinatal programme and hence applied to the entire parturient population.

Furthermore, a review of the obstetric services over the past 30 years leads us to the conclusion that there is an urgent need for detailed prospective evaluation studies to be carried out on many aspects of the maternity services; it is unsatisfactory to use retrospective observational data to establish causal relationships. As well as examining the outcome of pregnancy by traditional perinatal statistics, evaluation studies should take more account of consumer satisfaction by ensuring adequate feedback of information from patients. Public opinion surveys have found more adverse comments on the maternity services than any other branch of the National Health Service, and frequently these comments have arisen from areas of the country where the perinatal mortality is lowest. Concern has been expressed that recent trends in obstetric practice have unfairly placed the pregnant woman in the same category as the sick patient in other branches of medicine.

It is therefore timely to reflect on the objectives of an obstetric service. Since the majority of pregnant women enjoy an uncomplicated pregnancy and delivery, the main objectives of such a service should be: first, to ameliorate the minor discomforts of pregnancy and to prepare the couple for childbearing and child rearing; and second, to prevent, predict, recognize and manage factors that may affect the health of mother and child in that minority of pregnancies at risk. The knowledge, skills and attitudes required to achieve the first group of objectives are most likely to be found in community health personnel – namely, the family doctor, the health visitor and the community midwifery service – whereas the specialist obstetric services are most suited to deal with high risk patients. This concept provides the basis for a more rational use of non-specialist resources while allowing the specialist service to focus attention on those who are at greatest risk.

Little attempt has been made in the past to develop the use of predictors of potential perinatal risk. Most workers in this field have produced 'risk scores' based on assessment made in early pregnancy and again at the commencement of labour (13, 14). The allocation of weighted scores to each predictive factor to date has been purely empirical, and the potential risk of specific predictors either by themselves or in clusters will remain unknown until they are put to the test in clinical trials. More recently (15), scoring systems have been developed to assess pregnancy risk more specifically and independently, in terms of the three major causes of perinatal loss – (a) fetal congenital abnormality, (b) prematurity, and

(c) disorders of fetal growth in utero. By this technique a high risk population can be identified which will generate 75 per cent of perinatal deaths. It is estimated that about two-thirds of this high risk population are identifiable in early pregnancy and only an additional one-third would have to be recognized in late pregnancy or even in labour. Comprehensive prenatal and intrapartum fetal monitoring programmes could then be applied to the high risk groups, but the assessment of risk in early pregnancy allows a low risk population to be identified whose care should be the responsibility of the community obstetric service. It is assumed, of course, that this type of obstetric practice should be subject to rigorous evaluation.

As long as the role of the community obstetric service remains vague and undefined, it will probably continue to be the poor relation of the specialist hospital service. Yet, as well as being better equipped to meet the needs of the majority of pregnant women, the community service is also in a unique position to tackle some of the major problems confronting a modern maternity service. Its situation within the community could be used to launch a programme of pre-pregnancy assessment based on the assumption that sexually active couples within the reproductive age range fall into one of three groups: (a) those who do not want to become pregnant and hence require family planning advice; (b) those who are pregnant and have to be provided with prenatal care (there is, unfortunately, a substantial number of those whose pregnancy is unwanted and require emergency help with what is, in effect, a medical aid family emergency); (c) those who want to become pregnant and are consequently susceptible to advice on preparation for childbirth and child rearing (again, there is an unfortunate but substantial minority who will have difficulty in conceiving and will require special understanding and help). Such a pre-pregnancy assessment could include physical examination (especially assessment of blood pressure and urinalysis), cervical cytology, testing of immunity to rubella and an assessment of potential perinatal risk based on previous medical, obstetric and family history and also taking into account social indices of perinatal risk. Advice on smoking and obesity is likely to be more effective if counselling begins before conception. Furthermore, women in the high risk group, such as those with diabetes, hypertension or chronic renal disease, can be given the opportunity to discuss the principles of clinical management before embarking on a pregnancy.

The role of a community obstetric service in providing prenatal care requires to be revised in the light of the objectives outlined above. A programme of management should be based on a formal assessment of risk, clearly defined channels of referral for specialist advice, and expanded resources to extend the service more effectively to the lower socioeconomic groups. While being firmly of the opinion that universal hospital confinement in the UK will not reduce further the perinatal mortality, our limited resources dictate against the development of a comprehensive home delivery service. There is, therefore, a pressing need to review intrapartum patient care in maternity hospitals so as to make the service more acceptable to women and their families. This could be achieved by making provisions within hospitals for the delivery of low risk patients by a family doctor/midwife service linked to early discharge from hospital in the postnatal period.

Having considered the economic implications of the broad pattern of obstetric services, it is useful to cone down on the more restricted area of intrapartum care, and to consider all forms of obstetric intervention in terms of their benefits and costs. There are five specific forms of obstetric intervention in labour, all of which have come under public scrutiny – induction of labour, acceleration of labour by controlled infusion of oxytocic drugs, epidural analgesia for the relief of pain in labour, continuous fetal monitoring, and instrumental delivery of the baby. Each of these is a discrete operative procedure designed for a specific purpose, although they tend to be used collectively and may be regarded as interdependent. Thus, it would be a common practice to induce labour by amniotomy and oxytocin infusion, to monitor the uterine contractions and fetal heart rate continuously, to use an epidural anaesthetic to relieve the mother of pain, and to expedite delivery by the use of forceps. This has become part of general obstetric practice.

In reviewing the practice critically, it is salutary to consider the benefits and costs of each of these procedures. A consideration of postulated benefits presupposes a clear definition of the purposes of the procedure and some estimate of its efficiency in achieving these objectives.

Thus, the purpose of induction of labour may be to avoid the fetal hazards of a recognized complication of pregnancy, such as hypertension, Rhesus isoimmunization or antepartum haemorrhage. There are few obstetricians who would dispute the validity of this practice – indeed it forms the basis for the clinical management of these conditions. However, even within this area of medically indicated induction there is room for constant scrutiny. For example, the most common indication for induction is prolonged pregnancy – an ill-defined condition of poorly understood aetiology and epidemiology – and it is not unlikely that the risks of this condition are overdue for reappraisal. However, in all these situations the purpose of induction is to improve fetal survival and the benefits of induction must be measured by that yardstick. There may, however, be another category where induction is recommended for convenience – either of the patient or the maternity service. In these cases, it is against its efficiency in meeting this objective that the costs of induction must be balanced.

The purpose of acceleration of labour is to shorten the length of labour and thus to lessen the risks of uterine infection, reduce the duration of exposure of the fetus to the stress of labour, and decrease the period of discomfort for the mother – this can be measured either in terms of perinatal mortality and morbidity or in terms of maternal comfort. The purpose of epidural analgesia is primarily for the relief of pain, although it can sometimes be used to control maternal hypertension; consequently, epidural analgesia should be assessed by comparison with other traditional methods of pain relief. Continuous recording of the fetal heart rate, commonly used in conjunction with biochemical analysis of fetal blood obtained by scalp puncture, aims to provide a better index of fetal welfare in labour than that previously gained by intermittent auscultation – the goal is the elimination of intrapartum fetal asphyxia with avoidance of fetal death in utero and neonatal damage. Instrumental delivery includes caesarean section, forceps delivery and vacuum extraction – in general terms, these are designed to reduce fetal and maternal mortality and morbidity.

It is relatively easy to identify these objectives, but it has been difficult to measure the efficiency of these various procedures in achieving them. A common approach has been to study the outcome, usually in terms of crude perinatal mortality, comparing one control period of time followed by a subsequent test period when the procedure was introduced. This is open to the major fallacy that parturient populations change over the years – a serious problem today when widespread contraception, sterilization and abortion are almost eliminating grandmultiparity, illegitimacy, and pregnancy at the extremes of the reproductive age. An equally unacceptable alternative has been to compare different populations; for example, comparing two or three maternity hospitals and attributing observed differences in outcome to differences in practice.

It is clearly necessary to use either randomized control trials or alternative statistical techniques of multivariate analysis to isolate the effect of the procedure under study and eliminate other variables. Unfortunately, virtually no such studies have been performed, and it is consequently impossible to make an objective assessment of most forms of obstetric intervention – this is particularly unfortunate in the case of continuous fetal monitoring which has such widespread repercussions on obstetric practice. There is no clear evidence that its introduction has reduced perinatal mortality or morbidity. Similar statements apply to acceleration of labour. The assessment of induction of labour on 'non-medical' grounds is perhaps more difficult since its objectives are imprecise. Epidural anaesthesia is undoubtedly an effective method of pain relief for most women. Methods of instrumental delivery are an integral part of obstetric practice and have escaped critical evaluation. However, as caesarean section rates continue to rise and may exceed 15 per cent in some North American centres, it will be necessary constantly to assess that this intervention is at least achieving its objectives, however defined.

The costs of obstetric intervention are varied and substantial and may be considered in four categories. We are using the expression 'cost' here in the widest possible sense and not merely in financial terms, and we will agree that our analysis is tentative and incomplete.

1. *Direct costs to mother and child.* These include the immediate

adverse effects in terms of trauma, haemorrhage and infection. Maternal discomfort, short of physical damage, should also appear on the debit side. The risks of caesarean section and instrumental vaginal delivery, while substantially reduced in recent years, are still appreciable. In 1975 the incidence of sepsis in the puerperium was 1 per cent in patients delivered spontaneously and 14 per cent after an instrumental vaginal delivery or caesarean section in the Simpson Memorial Maternity Pavilion, Edinburgh. Haemorrhage in utero has occurred following scalp vein sampling in labour (16) but fortunately this complication is relatively infrequent. More commonly fetal monitoring is described as uncomfortable and can cause disquiet if not used sensitively and with careful explanation (17). Epidural analgesia is unfortunately not entirely without risk – these are, of course, minimized when used under expert control but could become a cause for concern if the service is inadequately supervised. Induction of labour is technically simple and in consequence is at risk of being used indiscriminately. It is salutary to recall that it carries the chance of unintentional premature delivery with all its attendant hazards, fetal asphyxia if oxytocin infusions are poorly controlled, and possibly an increase in recourse to caesarean section. It is not our intention to convey the idea that modern obstetrics is dangerous but that more intervention offers more opportunity for unintentional risk and that these must be actively sought out and examined and measured.

2. *Indirect costs to mother and child.* Current obstetric practice has indirect repercussions, some of which may be regarded as unfortunate for the family. Induction, acceleration and fetal monitoring all put constraints on the women in labour, introduce an element of intensive care to normal childbirth, and make it more difficult to achieve a friendly homely environment (16) – an approach well summed up in the phrase 'family centred obstetrics'. If one attaches importance to the participation of husband and family, it may be that a significant indirect cost of 'aggressive' obstetrics is the loss of this opportunity.

3. *Direct cost to society.* The financial costs of obstetric intervention are considerable. There will be considerable capital outlay in providing on a comprehensive national basis equipment for fetal monitoring and oxytocin infusion together with the costs of materials and maintenance. However, these are trivial in comparison with the cost of competent personnel to operate the equipment on a 24-hour basis. It should be observed that if it is done incompetently, giving unreliable or incorrect results, the hazards to the unfortunate patient are inexcusable. It is unfortunate that while an epidural service is an invaluable aid, it is also extremely expensive in terms of 24-hour specialist cover.

4. *Indirect costs to society.* This problem is compounded by the fact that any health service works within a finite budget and what is spent in one area inevitably limits one's ability to provide another type of service. It is in this context that one has to recognize that even within the restricted framework of reproductive medicine the cost of intrapartum intensive

care may prevent the development of other provisions for the community. If their benefits cannot be established beyond reasonable doubt, it may be that energy expended in some forms of obstetric practice would be better diverted, for example, to provide an improved vasectomy service or effective abortion counselling – two facilities which are poorly developed in the UK.

This discussion clearly reflects a concern with the trend of contemporary obstetric practice. It does not imply a retreat to therapeutic nihilism, but is critical of an unthinking acceptance of current professional fashions. There is clear evidence of some public concern with current obstetric practices and there is an overdue need for a reappraisal of their costs and benefits to society.

References

1. Baird, D. (1975). *British Journal of Preventive and Social Medicine,* **29**, 135.
2. Butler, N.R. and Alberman, E.D. (Editors) (1969). *Perinatal Problems.* Edinburgh and London, Churchill Livingstone.
3. Chamberlain, R. (Editor) (1970). *British Births.* London, Heinemann Medical.
4. Leading Article (1976). *British Medical Journal,* **2**, 729.
5. Cole, R.A., Howie, P.W. and Macnaughtone, M.C. (1975). *Lancet,* **1**, 767.
6. Chalmers, I., Ziosnikje, Johnska and Campbell, H. (1976). *British Medical Journal,* **1**, 735.
7. Peel, Sir John (Chairman) (1970). *Domiciliary Midwifery and Maternity Bed Needs.* Report of the Standing Maternity and Midwifery Advisory Committee. London, HMSO.
8. Abramowicz, H.C. and Richardson, S.E. (1975). *American Journal of Mental Deficiency,* **80**, 18.
9. Fairweather, D.V.I. and Illsley, R. (1960). *British Journal of Preventive and Social Medicine,* **14**, 149.
10. William, S. (1974). *British Medical Bulletin,* **30**, 252.
11. Hagard, S., Carter, F. and Milne, R.G. (1976). *British Journal of Preventive and Social Medicine,* **30**, 40.
12. Hagard, S. and Carter, F.A. (1976). *British Medical Journal,* **1**, 753.
13. Hobel, C.J., Hyvarinene, M.A., Okada, D.M. and Oh, W. (1973). *American Journal of Obstetrics and Gynecology,* **117**, 1.
14. Aubrey, R.H. and Pennington, J.C. (1973). *Clinical Obstetrics and Gynecology,* **16**, 3.
15. Boddy, K. and Parboosingh, J. (1977). Unpublished data.
16. Modanlou, H., Smith, E., Paul, R.H. and Hon, E.H. (1973). *Clinical Pediatrics,* **12**, 603.
17. Kitzinger, S. (1975). *Some Mothers' Experiences of Induced labour.* Submission to the Department of Health and Social Security from The National Childbirth Trust.

4

Paediatrics and Preventive Medicine

W. Morrice McCrae

Survival in childhood is now taken for granted. Parents in planning their families assume that all of their children will live. Parents' concern about the health of their children is not that they should live but that they should be free of handicaps or disabilities that might affect the quality of their lives. Paediatrics therefore has as its chief aim the prevention and mitigation of such handicaps, and the clinical practice of paediatrics is inseparable from preventive medicine. Success or failure of paediatrics is no longer reflected in mortality statistics. Success is the lessening of human misery which accompanies disease, and this cannot be easily measured or evaluated.

Although the human value of clinical paediatrics cannot be assessed, it must be acknowledged that the cost is high. Because of the increasingly high cost of the curative services in the National Health Service, preventive medicine is attracting new attention. The possibility is now being officially suggested (1) that if a greater share of the limited resources available were diverted to preventive medicine, this would in the long term effect savings in the expensive curative services.

This hypothesis is particularly difficult to examine in relation to paediatrics because the overlap between routine clinical practice and prevention is almost total. Nevertheless, there are a number of preventive measures which can be identified which clearly lie outside normal paediatric practice. In routine practice action is initiated by the parents seeking medical advice. Essentially, preventive practice may be thought of as those procedures initiated by the health services in the interest not only of individuals but of the community as a whole. These specifically preventive procedures will be considered not only in terms of their medical value, but also in relation to the question of whether their promotion is likely to reduce or increase the financial burdens of the National Health Service.

Antenatal Diagnosis

There are a number of ways in which the health of the child can be investigated before birth. Radiology can display the fetal skeleton, demonstrating not only bony abnormalities but also indicating the position and even numbers of the fetuses. By sonograph various parts, especially the head, can be measured. Fetal heart activity can be recorded by electrocardiography. Occasionally the fetus can be inspected directly, but to a limited extent, by fetoscopy. Biochemical investigations carried out on the mother's blood give very useful indications of placental function, and therefore indirectly of the state of the fetus. These techniques are used by obstetricians to ensure the birth of a normal child. They form part of preventive medicine only in so far as good obstetric practice is itself preventive medicine, a subject which will be discussed later.

However, antenatal diagnosis can also be carried out not to secure the birth of a normal child, but to prevent the birth of an abnormal one. If a serious and untreatable defect in the fetus can be detected before the 20th week of the pregnancy, the pregnancy can be terminated. The diagnosis is made by amniocentesis. By this technique fluid is drawn, by needle, from the sac surrounding the fetus. This is a safe procedure; the risk to mother and fetus is minimal. The examination is carried out at 14-15 weeks' gestation. At this time a satisfactory volume of fluid is available for testing, yet sufficient time remains to carry out the termination before 20 weeks when this is thought desirable.

More than 60 inherited disorders can be detected in this way. Most of these conditions are extremely rare, and although antenatal diagnosis is extremely valuable to the few families concerned, it is of little importance to the community. The few cases of these diseases which do occur represent no significant or even measurable financial charge on the NHS or burden on the community.

However, amniocentesis is now of considerable importance in the antenatal diagnosis of three relatively common types of disorder:

1. Down's syndrome (mongolism)
2. Malformations of the nervous system
3. Sex-linked conditions such as haemophilia

Down's Syndrome (Mongolism). This is a familiar condition in which there are a number of abnormalities, the most significant of which is mental deficiency. Compared with most inherited disorders it is quite common, occurring in 1 in 600 pregnancies. The prevalence is considerably affected by the age of the mother. In mothers under 20 years of age the prevalence is 0.54 per 1,000 births; over 40, it is 10.7 per 1,000. It can be readily diagnosed by the examination of the chromosomal pattern of the cells removed at amniocentesis. The diagnostic success rate has been estimated as high as 99 per cent. Theoretically, mongolism could therefore be prevented by examination of all pregnancies followed by abortion of all proven mongols. Such a programme would be extremely expensive. One study (2) concluded that if only the high risk group of mothers aged over 40 were examined, the cost of the investigation would be less than the potential cost of the care of the cases of mongolism prevented. However, if mothers younger than 40 were included, the financial benefit would progressively disappear as more mothers were subjected to investigation. Unfortunately, although the risk of mongolism in the pregnancies of mothers over 40 is relatively high, the number involved is small. If all pregnancies of mothers over 40 had been tested in Scotland in 1974 (i.e. 949) approximately 10 cases might have been prevented. During the same period 115 cases would have gone undetected in the many more pregnancies (i.e. 69,044) of younger mothers. In practice even the detection and prevention of 10 cases would be unlikely. Not all mothers in the older age group would present themselves at an antenatal clinic early enough in pregnancy to have this test carried out. Not all would have consented to termination and a large section of the community might find the whole concept repugnant.

Many centres make more limited use of the technique and examine only the pregnancies of mothers who have already had a mongol child, since the risk in a subsequent pregnancy is almost 2 per cent. This is an invaluable service to the mothers concerned, especially in relieving anxiety during the pregnancy. However, if the service were provided generally throughout the nation, cost benefit is unlikely since, without the service, mothers tend not to accept the risk and have no more children. The service would have little effect on the total number of mongol children to be cared for in the community.

Malformation of the Nervous System. In approximately 1 pregnancy in every 500 there is almost complete failure of development of the brain (anencephaly) and the child is either stillborn or dies within a few days of birth. In a similar number of pregnancies there are forms of incomplete development of the spinal cord (spina bifida) leading to variable, but often severe, physical handicap. Where spina bifida is associated with hydrocephalus there may be mental handicap as well. The delivery of such affected infants causes extreme distress to the families and when the child survives with severe handicap, the continuing burden on the parents is very great.

In most such cases there is no continuing burden on the health services. All of the cases of anencephaly are either stillborn or die within days of delivery, and only 47 per cent of cases of spina bifida survive to the age of 1 year. Until recently it was the usual practice to attempt surgical treatment in almost all cases of spina bifida. It is now becoming accepted that there should be strict criteria of selection of neonates for surgery. As a result the number of survivors, particularly survivors with severe handicap, is falling. However, the treatment of even this reduced number of survivors is expensive. In a study in the Western Regional Hospital Board (Scotland) in 1973 it was estimated that the lifetime cost of caring for the spina bifida cases born in that region alone in one year, would be more than £1 million.

In 1972 it was shown that in the presence of anencephaly the amniotic fluid contained high levels of alpha-feto protein (AFP). In 1973 this was found also to be the case in open cases of spina bifida. Subsequently, the accuracy of this test on fluid obtained by amniocentesis during the second trimester has been shown to be high. It has therefore become customary to offer this test to all pregnant women who have previously borne an affected child, since their pregnancies are known to be ten times more at risk than the average. The assurance that a recurrence of the abnormality can be detected and the pregnancy terminated where necessary is of great comfort to these mothers, but in the community the effect is small. If there were universal acceptance of amniocentesis and termination by all women in this high risk group, only a 10 per cent reduction in the overall prevalence of spina bifida at birth would be achieved, and this at considerable cost.

Because of the cost involved there has been no serious proposal that all pregnancies should be screened by amniocentesis. However, a more recent discovery has led to a reassessment of the possibility of at least a degree of screening (3). In 1974 it was reported that there was an association between raised alpha-feto protein levels in the mother's blood and the presence of a fetus with a neural tube defect. This simple blood test is usually acceptable to the patient and is very much cheaper to carry out than amniocentesis. It is therefore possible that this blood test might form the basis of a universal screening programme. It is proposed that the maternal blood should be tested for AFP as part of routine antenatal care in every pregnancy. If a raised level were found, then the mother would be offered amniocentesis for confirmation of the diagnosis and termination carried out as indicated.

The cost effectiveness of such a scheme is difficult to calculate. At present the chief difficulty is the lack of agreement on the sensitivity of the blood test. Optimistically, a single blood test has been claimed to be positive in 80 per cent of affected pregnancies; others have suggested a sensitivity of only 20 per cent. The study by Hagard and his colleagues presents interesting forecasts. Given that 90 per cent of women attend an antenatal clinic at the appropriate time; given total co-operation by the patients; given a sensitivity of 80 per cent for the blood test: 75 out of 120 pregnancies affected by spina bifida annually in their region could be detected and terminated. The economic benefits given these conditions were calculated to outweigh costs in the ratio 1.86:1. This study is open to criticism on a number of grounds. It may be that the attendance rate of 90 per cent is over-optimistic. The readiness of the patients to opt for termination may also be exaggerated to an important extent.

However, in the absence of reliable figures, the assumptions on attendance and acceptability may perhaps be allowed to stand for the sake of argument, even though they are probably too high. But the results of the study certainly must be reassessed in the light of accumulating experience of the sensitivity of the screening blood test. This has proved to be 90 per cent for anencephaly but as low as 40 per cent for spina bifida. By their own calculation at this reduced sensitivity this scheme would have a benefit cost index of only 0.7.

It therefore appears that universal screening for spina bifida by measuring AFP in maternal blood could result in some reduction, perhaps by 25 per cent in the total number of surviving patients, but there would be no cost benefit.

Sex-linked Disorders. Perhaps the best known condition of this type is haemophilia. The abnormality is carried on the X chromosome. Females may therefore be carriers of the gene but remain unaffected. Only males are affected.

There is at present no certain method of detecting carriers. However, some women become known to be carriers because of the birth of an affected son. Others may be suspected of being carriers because of a family history of haemophilia. When pregnant, these carriers can now be offered amniocentesis. Although it is not possible to diagnose haemophilia in the fetus, it is easy to determine the sex. If the fetus is male, there is a 50 per cent chance that it will be affected by haemophilia. If the fetus is female, it cannot be affected but there is a 50 per cent chance of its being a carrier. By aborting all the males in such pregnancies the birth of a haemophiliac infant would be prevented. The cost effectiveness of such a practice would be very satisfactory.

There are certain limitations which must be mentioned. The number of affected male fetuses aborted would be equalled by the number of quite normal fetuses aborted. Some may find this unacceptable. In addition, should the parents decide to proceed to have the same number of children that they would have planned if they had not known of the risk of haemophilia, the action to ensure that all their children were girls would have the eventual effect of increasing the number of carriers in the community. The attempt to keep the family free of haemophilia would necessitate an ever increasing number of abortions in succeeding generations including more and more carriers unless some reliable method of detecting carriers is found.

Amniocentesis widely performed and the results acted upon could greatly reduce the incidence of haemophilia from the present level of 6:100,000 but new spontaneous mutations would always prevent the total elimination of the disease.

Amniocentesis – Conclusion. Amniocentesis is proving an extremely useful technique in preventive medicine. It is too costly to be considered for universal screening. However, when the clinician recognizes that his patient is at particular risk of having a child affected by mongolism, spina bifida, haemophilia or certain other, much less common, metabolic or chromosomal disorders, amniocentesis has now become an essential investigation. Distress and suffering can be greatly lessened. However, even when 'at risk' patients are carefully selected, no overall financial saving will be achieved by the introduction of this technique.

Screening

Short of true prevention, there are obvious attractions in detecting defects at an early stage when they have done little harm, and may be relatively easy to correct.

'Population screening' is the carrying out of some test or procedure in every member of a population (e.g. all newborn, all school leavers) to detect unrecognized defect or disease.

In 'at risk screening' the test or procedure is carried out only on a limited number of selected subjects for whom there is already some medical reason to suspect that they may be affected. For example, if one child in a family is found to have tuberculosis or Wilson's disease (an inherited metabolic disease causing liver damage), it would be normal practice to test his siblings. This form of screening is naturally much more productive in the number of cases found than population screening. However, at risk screening will not be considered here because it forms part of normal clinical practice. Our chief concern is with population screening.

The neonatal period offers an almost ideal opportunity for such screening. Obviously it offers the ultimate potential in early diagnosis of inherited or congenital disorders. There is also the great practical advantage that the population is easily accessible for investigation since almost all deliveries are now in hospital.

Childhood populations again become available for screening when at school and certain screening procedures can be carried out on school entry or on leaving.

Screening at other ages is less easy. Preschool children are difficult to reach and any screening programme is very dependent for success on the promotion of publicity and the persuasion of mothers to co-operate.

Neonatal Screening. It is particularly difficult in the neonatal period to distinguish between 'prevention' and routine practice. All newborn are weighed. This is a form of screening in itself, since it detects those small infants in need of special nursing and medical care. About 6 per cent of all infants have some congenital abnormality. Many of these are detected by physical examination by a clinician in the first day of life. The best documented example of the preventive effect of physical examination of the newborn is the detection of congenital dislocation of the hip. This abnormality affects rather more than 1 in 1,000 children. It first makes itself obvious when the child learns to walk and his gait is seen to be abnormal. Operative treatment at this late stage is difficult and results are not always satisfactory. Fortunately, the defect can be detected in the newborn period during routine examination. An experienced clinician may be expected to achieve some 90 per cent success in detection. If the diagnosis is made in the neonatal period the only, but effective, treatment required is splinting in abduction for some weeks.

The principal laboratory screening programme being carried out in the UK in the neonatal period is for the detection of cases of phenylketonuria (PKU). This is a clearly defined metabolic abnormality which leads to mental deficiency. The incidence is approximately 1 in 20,000. Unfortunately, there is some regional variation in incidence. Local doubts about the exact incidence detracts from the certainty that the programme is fully efficient since there is no exact 'expected' number to be compared with the actual number detected. There is also some variation in severity. Most untreated cases are incapable of independent existence because of their mental defect. However, research screening of adults has indicated that 1 in 80,000 of the general population have the abnormality and are able to support themselves although of low intellectual ability. This leads to uncertainty in assessing how much has been achieved in treating any single case. Nevertheless, the general efficacy of treatment is beyond doubt (4). Treatment is dietary and must be continued for 10 years, but to be effective is must be instituted very soon after birth.

The screening is carried out on the sixth day of life. A drop of blood is collected on to filter paper which is sent by post to a central laboratory. The laboratory test is not expensive. It is sensitive (i.e. it detects a very high percentage of affected cases) and has a high specificity (i.e. there are few false positives).

The programme is ethically justifiable in that the subjects screened suffer no harm and the affected subjects benefit. Scientifically, it is satisfactory in that the test is efficient and the effect of treatment has been measured. The programme has also improved knowledge of the incidence and range of severity of the disease.

Carter (5) has estimated the cost of detection of each single case at £6,000. The cost of treatment has been estimated at £30,000 over 10 years, and, including the cost of medical care and follow-up, the total cost of preventing one case of mental deficiency is approximately £37,000. However, this has to be set against the saving in institutional care for each patient for perhaps 30 years. In this estimate that cost would be £46,800.

It is concluded that screening for PKU is worthwhile (6) in that it is ethically, scientifically and financially justifiable. However, the number of patients rescued and treated is small, perhaps 4 each year in Scotland. The total effect on the incidence of mental deficiency is minimal.

The sample of blood taken for the detection of PKU can be examined for the presence of other metabolic abnormalities, none of which would justify a screening programme of its own. Galactosaemia has an incidence of 1 in 40,000 but in most cases it is usually clinically evident before the sixth day when the test is taken. Only mild or atypical cases would be diagnosed as a result of screening. Maple syrup urine disease, homocystinuria, tyrosinaemia can also be detected. These abnormalities are extremely rare, so rare that their exact incidence is unknown. For that reason, as well as the uncertainty and difficulty of treatment, screening is not justified.

Screening for PKU is a success, although the disease itself is rare. It would clearly be desirable to devise similar programmes for more common diseases.

Cystic fibrosis illustrates some of the difficulties in such projects. Cystic fibrosis is the commonest inherited metabolic disease, with an incidence of 1 in 2,000. Screening may be possible and programmes of universal screening are being considered. It is known that at birth the meconium in cases of cystic fibrosis contains abnormally high amounts of protein and this can be detected by the midwife using a simple and inexpensive strip test. The number of false positives is rather high and there are some false negatives. The test is therefore not diagnostic and the tentative diagnosis from screening has to be confirmed by measurement of the concentration of sodium and chloride in sweat. This test is very reliable but is too elaborate and time consuming to be used as a screening test. It has been estimated that 60 per cent of cystic fibrosis could be detected by the screening test for protein in meconium followed by a sweat test.

Cystic fibrosis, however, is a poorly understood condition. It is recognized clinically by the association of recurring pulmonary infection with malabsorption due to pancreatic deficiency and certain other less important abnormalities. The cause is unknown and the condition therefore cannot be defined. There is a wide variation in severity, some dying in infancy, others reaching well into adult life. In 1 in every 400 cases of clinical cystic fibrosis the sweat test (usually regarded as diagnostic) is normal. There are also many people who have abnormal sweat sodium concentrations with no other evidence of cystic fibrosis. If a case of cystic fibrosis were detected by screening, it would therefore be impossible to say exactly what had been detected in terms of pathology and prognosis. In addition, there is no definitive treatment for cystic fibrosis. Care is only supportive. The effectiveness of treatment is variable and there is no evidence that early treatment, begun before symptoms appear, improves the prognosis. Cases detected by screening cannot be assured of benefit from early detection and if an unduly bad prognosis is given, their morale and their lives generally may be unduly and even unnecessarily harmed.

Screening for cystic fibrosis, although possible, is not justifiable either scientifically or ethically.

Financially the situation is uncertain. The cost of detecting each case would exceed £10,000. Treatment presumably would begin earlier as the result of screening and early diagnosis; otherwise screening is pointless.

There is no certainty that this would affect the ultimate prognosis but, if early treatment had any effect, this should be to prolong the period of life during which supportive treatment is required. Hospital admissions during the later and more severe stages of the disease would be delayed but not prevented. The financial result would inevitably be an increase in the total cost of treatment.

Because a possible method for screening exists there is a temptation to use it. But this temptation should be resisted unless benefit can be demonstrated either to the individual or to the community. That is not the case in cystic fibrosis.

Health Surveillance

Screening in Preschool Children. There are many proponents of the idea that children should be examined at intervals during growth and development as an important component of primary medical care, the objective being the early detection and amelioration of handicap.

Unlike neonates and school children, preschool children are not a 'captive' population. Any organization set up specifically for screening would have difficulties in finding and gaining access to the population to be screened. A possible solution is for general practitioners to screen the children in their own practices. This was attempted in Livingston New Town in 1972 by a group of six doctors, including two with extensive postgraduate experience of paediatrics (7). The children were examined at the ages of 6 weeks, 6 months, 16 months, 3 years and 4½ years. (This general practice has the unusual advantage of a computer assisted records system.)

Children were sent three appointments at each of these ages. If they still did not attend a health visitor visited the family to add further persuasion. An overall acceptance rate of 73 per cent was achieved.

The children were examined for those abnormalities included in the Scottish Home and Health Department's list of handicapping conditions and for behaviour disorders. At total of 1,204 children were examined; 82 abnormalities were found, of which 76 had already been recognized and recorded. Only 6 abnormalities (1 coeliac, 1 mental handicap, 1 case of deafness, 1 case of Werdnig-Hoffmann's disease, 1 dislocated hip and 1 expressive dysphasia) were detected for the first time by screening, and not all of these are treatable.

A somewhat similar study (8) was carried out at the Woodside Health Centre, Glasgow (under the direction of the Professor of General Practice and again in practices with excellent resources). A three-tier system was used. The initial examination was by a doctor and a health visitor, or, in some examinations by a health visitor alone. Cases of possible abnormality were referred to a local authority assessment centre. Thereafter, if doubts still remained the child was referred for specialist opinion.

Examinations were carried out at 6 weeks, 6 months, 10 months, 18 months, 2 years, 3 years and 4½ years. The report is almost entirely about their experience of children up to the age of 18 months. The overall acceptance rate, after two offered appointments and at least one visit by a health visitor, was 76.3 per cent. Defaulting increased from 14.5 per cent at 6 weeks to 39.7 per cent at 18 months. There were 475 children in the scheme. Five abnormalities were found: 1 mongol at 6 weeks; a cyanotic congenital heart disease, multiple congenital abnormalities at 6 months; 2 hearing defects at 10 months. As the authors concede, it is impossible to be sure that any of these children actually benefited, but the two diagnoses of deafness were probably useful.

These two studies were performed in practices which are unusually well staffed and equipped. So little has been achieved by these programmes that general practitioners with lesser resources are not likely to be encouraged to undertake such developmental screening in their practices. Perhaps there are hidden benefits. It may be that the reassurance provided to the mothers involved prevented a number of unnecessary consultations at other times. This can only be speculation. There seems very little evidence of substantial benefit and certainly no cost benefit from developmental screening, but further study is required. Meantime, one must be impressed, from the results of the Livingston Study, by the ability of the parents to detect abnormal signs in the physical and mental development of the preschool child and to obtain the appropriate medical care.

Selective Screening. If, as seems likely, repeated developmental screening during the preschool years is not worthwhile, there may yet be a place for selective screening for specific important defects carried out on one occasion only. The relevant defects would be those least likely to be suspected by the parents. Two such defects have been subjects of trials of selective screening: hearing defects and visual defects.

It is important that hearing defects should be detected early before speech development is seriously prejudiced. Few would doubt the value of early diagnosis. The value of early diagnosis of squints and other ocular defects is less clear, but is probably desirable.

The detection of hearing and ocular defects at the age of 2 or 3 years is possible (9, 10) but a screening programme would present difficulties. The necessary techniques are difficult and require considerable expertise. This in itself implies expense, and the need for a publicity campaign to attract the interest of parents would add to the costs. Active co-operation from parents would be required and the response rate especially in the most needy families is difficult to forecast.

Trials of screening of preschool children would be required to assess response rate, benefit and cost before selective screening could be advocated. Benefit to the children is quite possible. The cost would be great and no long-term cost benefit to the National Health Service can be foreseen.

Screening of School Children. School children form a very convenient population for screening purposes since they are so readily available for study. It is generally agreed that it is important that defects such as undescended testes, hearing and speech and reading defects and growth abnormalities should be detected. School medical examinations have been carried out for many years, for which the cost of medical manpower must be enormous. It is strange therefore that D'Souza (11) should be able to complain, in a journal issued by the Chief Medical Officer of the Scottish Home and Health Department, that there has never been any serious appraisal of the methods employed in detecting abnormalities in school children and, in particular, whether present screening methods are appropriate. The records show how many abnormalities were found at school medical examinations. However, it is impossible to tell how many of these abnormalities were already known, what treatment was arranged and, in effect, how much the children benefited from having their abnormalities examined. On the other hand, in a recent survey Vimpani (12) examined 48,000 school children specifically for small stature. Thirty-two cases were found, all resulting from correctable pathology, but undetected by previous school examination. It may be that screening for defects by general physical examination, especially when conducted by medical officers with few other medical activities, becomes so tedious it also becomes inefficient.

School medical examinations have always been accepted as desirable. The recently published Court Report (13) clearly indicates that it is to be government policy to increase the resources devoted to this type of health surveillance. In 1973, 3,250 doctors were already employed either part-time or full-time by the local authorities for clinical work in the child health and school health services in England and Wales. A further 1,648 GPs were employed on a part-time basis. Health surveillance is therefore expensive and about to become more so. It is possible that expanded and better child health services following the Court Report may improve the lot of numbers of children but it is impossible to foresee, other than that the overall cost of the NHS will be increased.

Case Finding

The Livingston Study already quoted indicates parents' ability to detect disorders in their young children. In later childhood this pattern persists. Idiopathic scoliosis in adolescent girls is a good illustration. This abnormality is potentially crippling. If neglected it may proceed to gross chest deformity with resultant respiratory difficulty and even respiratory failure. Although it is also common, affecting 2 per 1,000, there is no drive by orthopaedic surgeons to have screening programmes, such is their confidence that the defect is always noticed early and cases reach an orthopaedic surgeon at a treatable stage.

Most parents make full use of medical services where they are available. In a study in south-east Scotland (13) it was found that 1 in 6 of the childhood population was seen by a paediatrician each year. Many of these referrals were for trivial reasons or for purposes of reassurance about specific anxieties. However, no matter the nature of the presenting problem; examination of the child includes developmental screening. The potential for case finding by paediatricians in their everyday practice is therefore enormous. In evaluating any new programme for prevention of handicap by the early detection of disease by screening, it is also essential to assess the probability that the disease would be detected by parents, practitioner or paediatrician in the normal course of events. This probability will vary in different parts of the country and in different social groups.

Control of Infectious Disease

No medical procedure has a better cost/benefit ratio than immunization against the formerly common childhood infectious diseases. Poliomyelitis provides a good example. The saving in medical and other costs over the past 20 years has been more than twelve times the cost of the immunization programme. In spite of this example, it does not follow that all available forms of immunization should be universally promoted. Indeed, such a practice could be counter-productive.

It must be appreciated that factors other than immunity affect the incidence of infectious disease. Most important of these is improvement in living standards. It has often been shown that the incidence of infectious disease was already falling years before any adequate medical treatment or immunization was availablve. Between 1900 and 1960 the mortality from measles fell from 30 to 0.1 per 100,000 of the population with no immunization. This effect continues. The incidence of scarlet fever, for which there is no form of immunization, has been falling parallel with that of whooping cough for which immunization has been widely used.

Classically, the basic methods of coping with infection have been to eradicate the source and interfere with spread. These methods have been particularly successful with bacterial infections and the degree of success which can be achieved is illustrated by the virtual eradication of tuberculosis. Immunization of the subjects at risk is the third line of defence, and its importance will vary according to the size of that risk.

The value of immunization must therefore be kept continually under review. The factors involved can be illustrated by the case of vaccination against smallpox. This disease has not been endemic in Britain since 1935; smallpox in this country is always imported. In the 20 years up to 1973, there were 13 importations leading to 103 local cases and 37 deaths. The fact that these importations were well contained is not attributable to an immunity of the population conferred by immunization, since over the same period only 10 per cent of the population were effectively vaccinated. The containment of the infection was the result of successful isolation of cases and the vaccination and surveillance of contacts. The low rate of immunity of the population is of interest. Primary vaccination is received by only 40 per cent of the population. Although revaccination is required every 3 years this is only carried out in about 10 per cent. This low acceptance rate of vaccination is probably due to an appreciation of the balance of risks.

Vaccination itself carries some risk: from encephalitis, chronic progressive vaccinia and eczema vaccinatum. It has been calculated that, at present rates of vaccination, 150 deaths could be expected from these complications between 1971 and 2000. This is approximately the same number of deaths that could be expected from 50 importations of smallpox into the country over the same period. This number of importations is most unlikely. First, the number of importations in recent years has been very much less than this figure and, more important, the number of sources of infection is progressively being reduced. Smallpox is now endemic only in Ethiopia, the Sudan, India, Pakistan and Nepal. There is a very good prospect that this reservoir of infection will be even further reduced. As a result, the position has now been reached in Britain that, with the possible exception of doctors and other health workers, vaccination represents a greater risk than the smallpox which it aims to prevent.

Immunization against whooping cough is under scrutiny for slightly different reasons. It is known that minor febrile reactions after the injection are common. More serious reactions leading to permanent brain damage also occur but are rare. In the past these risks have been accepted because of the severity of whooping cough itself. However, disease can vary not only in incidence, like scarlet fever or smallpox; it can also vary in severity. There is now some indication that whooping cough is a milder disease than it was, presenting a real danger only to very young infants. The current practice of immunization at the age of 6 months has the result of leaving unprotected the only age group which would materially benefit from protection. Many believe that in these circumstances the risk of immunization is no longer acceptable. Unfortunately, if the trend to withhold immunization in the interests of the individual continues and the number of protected children declines, then the 'herd' immunity of the population as a whole may also fall to an extent that will materially increase the risks of whooping cough.

This problem is unresolved, but the controversy it has aroused may prove useful in drawing attention to the need to keep immunization practice under constant review. Unfortunately, informed discussion is generally confined to medical and ministerial circles. The public is influenced largely by rumour. Uncertainty and anxiety are the results.

Immunization is a cheap and effective weapon against infectious disease, but it is useless unless accepted by the population at risk. Doubts about whooping cough tend to spill over and unjustifiably affect other immunizations such as diphtheria, and acceptance rates fall. Much more must be spent on informing the public of the benefits and explaining the nature of the hazards. A better informed public might be expected to respond to variations in immunization policy made desirable by change in circumstance.

Conclusion

The 'preventive' value of good clinical practice cannot be doubted. The fall in the perinatal mortality rate is the result of good obstetric practice and reduction in mortality is paralleled by reduction in fetal damage and resultant handicap. The number of handicaps thus prevented enormously outnumber those defects which are inherited, and are made the subject of elaborate screening tests carried out on neonates.

Similarly, the disorders of childhood detected by parents, general practitioners and paediatricians in the normal course of events greatly outnumber the few detected only as the result of 'screening' medical examination in the course of health surveillance.

There is great need therefore for programmes of 'prevention' to be evaluated. Improvement in living standards is generally acknowledged as the major influence on child health. In a sense the benefit could be regarded as without cost since the improvements are desirable in themselves and the public would probably regard the effect on health as merely an additional bonus.

Other deliberate alterations in the environment such as fluoridation of the water supply would clearly be highly cost effective.

However, when schemes of prevention aim not to affect the population as a whole, but to detect and ameliorate the defects and diseases of individuals there can be no assumption of cost benefit. Each individual scheme must be assessed separately. The probability is that in many instances it will be found that prevention is possible but costly. Like improved treatment, improved prevention, however desirable, will often be an expense rather than a saving.

References

1. DHSS (1976). *Prevention and Health: Everybody's Business.* London, HMSO.
2. Hagard, S. and Carter, F.A. (1976). *British Medical Journal,* **1**, 753.
3. Hagard, S., Carter, F.A. and Milne, R.G. (1976). *British Journal of Preventive and Social Medicine,* **30**, 40.
4. Dobson, F.K., Williamson, M. and Friedman, F.G. (1976). *Pediatrics,* **58**, 53.
5. Carter, F.A. (1976). *Journal of the Royal College of Physicians,* **10**, 153.
6. Cochrane, A.L. and Holland, W.W. (1971). *British Medical Bulletin,* **47**, 3.
7. Bain, D.J.G. (1974). *Health Bulletin,* Scottish Home and Health Department.
8. Farber, J.H., Boothman, R. and Stansfield, G.P. (1976). *Health Bulletin,* Scottish Home and Health Department.

9. Oliver, H. (1971). *British Journal of Ophthalmology,* **55**, 462.
10. Blair, F. (1961). *Exceptional Children,* **36**, 259.
11. D'Souza, M.F. (1976). *Health Bulletin,* Scottish Home and Health Department.
12. Vimpani, D. (1977). Personal communication.
13. *Fit for the Future* (1977). Report of the Committee on Child Health Services. London, HMSO.

5

The Cost of Rescue and the Price of Survival

Bryan Jennett

'It is silliness to live when to live is torment;
And then have we a prescription to die
When death is our physician.'
Othello, Act I, scene iii

'... immediate needs will get priority over anticipatory care, and dramatic though possibly ineffective episodic care will win out in confrontation with the demands of primary care and care of the chronic sick and handicapped.'
J.T. Hart (1)

'... there is too much unjustified therapy — placebos, rituals, defensive manoeuvres to avoid a courageous judgement. The NHS should stand only for treatment that is rationally and humanely justified.'
R. Maxwell of McKinsey and Co (2)

Death provides a ready measure of the outcome of illness. Mortality rates and survival times are common yardsticks by which doctors assess therapy for life-threatening conditions. Faced with such illness, patients and their families naturally hope that doctors will succeed in averting or postponing death. Society's interest is less with individual deaths than with the reassurance that comes from witnessing reasonable efforts being made to save lives, even if these are not always successful. Inevitably therefore doctors in acute hospitals spend a good deal of time and effort trying to rescue patients from death. With the increasing availability and effectiveness of technological means of prolonging life, doubts are sometimes expressed about the appropriateness of using them routinely. This is partly because of concern about the quality and duration of life after life-saving interventions in some circumstances; and partly because of the increasing cost of these procedures, both in absolute terms and as a proportion of the resources expended in the acute hospital sector.

What are Rescue Procedures?

When discussing the relative proportions of time, space, staff and equipment which are devoted to different activities in acute hospitals a distinction is often made between cure and care. It is helpful to recognize a third type of activity, namely *rescue* (3). Rescue procedures are frequently successful in restoring patients to relative health, at least temporarily, and sometimes a cure is achieved. More often the result of 'successful' rescue is to prolong, or to create, a need for prolonged care. The interaction and balance between these three aspects of the acute hospital services is therefore complex.

Rescue procedures relate to life and death situations, in that if intervention is withheld the patient can be expected to die in the near future. They include many procedures in the fields of intensive care, oncology, renal dialysis and transplantation, intracranial surgery, open heart surgery and neonatal surgery. These involve special facilities which are usually available only on a regional basis and are therefore very susceptible to control by resource allocation, because if treatment cannot be provided at the specified centre there is no alternative. Another characteristic of the conditions which require rescue therapy is that rapid, if not immediate, intervention is often required.

Examples of Rescue Procedures

Renal Dialysis and Transplantation. These are of proved effectiveness in prolonging good quality of life in certain clear-cut circumstances. There have never been enough dialysis machines or cadaver kidneys to treat all the patients who might benefit, and consequently rules of selection of patients for treatment have had to be evolved. The costs of treatment, of the relative benefits of dialysis and transplantation, and of the consequences of withholding treatment have all been well worked out. This field of activity therefore provides a good example of how to deal with allocating restricted resources for rescue treatment.

Congenital Abnormalities. The spina bifida controversy has been widely reported in recent years and need not be recounted in detail (4). Dispute centres on the worst affected babies, who previously were never offered treatment of any kind. There then emerged the recommendation that emergency surgical closure of the spinal defect was essential, within 48 hours of birth; shunting procedures for hydrocephalus were usually required either at this time or shortly afterwards. Survivors often faced permanent paraplegia and required a series of urological and orthopaedic operations as well as repeated ventricular shunts for the control of hydrocephalus. Few of these permanently crippled children had normal intelligence, and many families were devastated by the need to provide continuing care; in time special schools and permanent institutional care became necessary for some survivors. More recently it has become more acceptable to undertake careful assessment of the probable ultimate outcome before embarking on initial treatment, in the hope of identifying those in whom the outlook is expected to be bad and to withhold treatment from such babies. Although there remain differences of detail about the exact criteria, and about the best course to be followed for those from whom treatment is withheld, there are few surgeons or paediatricians who still advocate operating on all affected babies. This story provides a good example of the consequences, both financial and in suffering, when elaborate rescue measures are enthusiastically promoted without having been subjected to a controlled trial which included assessment of benefit and cost in the broadest sense, and in the long as well as the short term.

Severe Head Injuries. It is 20 years since it was reported that the mortality rate from these injuries could be halved by the use of intensive respiratory care (5). Since then various other procedures, including early decompression and prolonged periods of controlled ventilation, have been recommended. However, reported mortality appears to be similar among injuries of comparable severity differently treated, whilst a proportion of the patients whose lives are saved remain so severely disabled that they are dependent for the rest of their lives (6). Again the problem is to recognize the potential for recovery soon enough after injury to influence the decision to institute active therapy or to discontinue life-support measures. Similar considerations apply also to other forms of acute brain damage, such as those due to cardiorespiratory arrest and spontaneous intracranial haemorrhage (5).

Oncology. The treatment of malignant disease poses challenges for surgeons, radiotherapists and chemotherapists – as well as for the patient, the family and the family doctor. Striking success can be claimed for each of these methods of treatment, alone or in combination, in the management of certain tumours, provided they have not already spread too far. Unfortunately, there are still many tumours which careful studies show to have been scarcely affected in their natural history by any available method of treatment. In others the gains are marginal in terms of the quality and duration of survival, so that it is doubtful whether the effort expended by therapeutic teams, and the discomfort and hazards suffered by patients, make it justifiable to have embarked on treatment at all.

The diagnosis of cancer has such serious implications that there is an understandable compulsion to embark immediately on elaborate treatment.

As a consequence there is probably more unjustifiable therapeutic endeavour in this field than in any other. Massive abdominal resections are sometimes carried out when it is obvious that the tumour is inoperable, and even when it is unlikely that any palliative benefit can be expected to result. For years victims of breast cancer were subjected to the mutilation of radical mastectomy which controlled trials now often show to have no advantage over simpler procedures. Much of the radiotherapy carried out for gliomas of the brain and for carcinoma of the bronchus is little more than an expensive placebo. There is a considerable risk that chemotherapy, so strikingly successful in childhood leukaemia, may begin to be used relatively indiscriminately for progressive malignancy, particularly as it requires relatively limited supporting services when used in dosages which are not toxic – and which are therefore probably relatively ineffective. Some of the muddle in this field arises from failure to distinguish between treatment designed to produce symptomatic palliation, and that which aims to prolong survival and to control tumour growth. Increasing interest in the overall management of the dying patient, including the control of pain and the sympathetic handling of the patient and his family, promises to lead to a more realistic assessment of the goals and achievements of treatment for malignant disease which cannot be cured; it is hoped that there may then be less compulsion to employ inappropriate aggressive measures in the name of palliation. The counter-argument to such a view is to point out that in the early days of chemotherapy for leukaemia few patients were cured, and many suffered from the effects of treatment which failed to cure them; yet the doctors pressed on. That was, however, in the context of well controlled trials – which is the only ethical justification for employing measures that show promise but are not yet established, especially if they are expensive and hazardous.

Assessing Outcome After Rescue

The result of rescue depends on many factors but the most important determinant is usually the underlying condition. Expensive and expeditious intervention may achieve a result which is satisfactory in the short term but the underlying disease process soon leads to relapse, which is often fatal. This is most obviously the case when a crisis occurs in a patient with chronic, progressive organ failure (e.g. respiratory, cardiac, hepatic), but it applies also to many patients in coma or with malignant disease. In such conditions it is necessary to record not only whether death was averted in the short term but also what the ultimate outcome was. In one large series of patients with non-traumatic coma (excluding poisoning), of those alive at 1 month, 57 per cent were dead at 12 months, an overall mortality of 89 per cent (7). Of patients requiring intensive therapy after elective surgery for neoplastic disease in one unit, only 6 per cent were alive at 1 year; of 226 patients requiring intensive physician and nursing care, 73 per cent were dead a year later, and only 12 per cent were restored to their pre-illness state (8). By contrast, patients admitted to the same unit for routine postoperative monitoring had 90 per cent survival at 1 year. This emphasizes how important an influence admission criteria (i.e. patient selection) can have on the results of treatment, especially of rescue.

In survivors in a general intensive care unit, mental function recovers far better than physical capacity. When rescue achieves survival after severe brain damage the opposite is the case, mental disability contributing much more significantly to the overall social outcome (9). Those with marked physical disability due to brain damage almost always have some impairment of personality and memory, whilst many patients who have made a good physical recovery prove to have considerable changes in mental function; unless outcome is assessed critically the latter cases are easily misjudged as being more fully recovered than they really are. A simple scale by which to judge this social outcome after brain damage has been described (10) which has proved useful in practice. Four categories of survival are recognized: the vegetative state (11); the severely disabled (conscious but dependent); the moderately disabled (independent but disabled); and good recovery. What level on this scale should be regarded as an acceptable result of treatment is obviously a value judgement – and that will depend on who is the judge.

An attempt has been made to test opinion about states of survival after brain damage by asking groups of people to record anonymously which they consider to be worse, for the patient and also for the family, of two pairs of outcome – death or vegetative survival, and vegetative survival or severe disability. This was asked of 130 senior health professionals and lawyers attending a meeting on severe brain damage in San Francisco; a week later it was administered to 130 medical students who were in their first year of clinical studies in Glasgow. In spite of the wide difference in age and experience the response were very similar. About 90 per cent regarded vegetative survival as worse than death both for the patient and the family. Over 40 per cent considered that to regain consciousness, but to be dependent, would be worse than the vegetative state for the patient himself; but less than 20 per cent of respondents thought the family would think this. Subsequent surveys among nurses and general practitioners in Britain, and among nurses and students in the Netherlands, show a similar pattern. This kind of questionnaire approach can be criticized on philosophical and theoretical grounds; but the consistency of the response makes it difficult to escape the conclusion that many people are now willing to admit that survival after severe brain damage may be judged a disaster for the victim and his family. It is the combination of mental impairment with physical handicap that makes disability after brain damage so devastating, not only for the patient but for the family who, especially if the patient has limited insight, may bear most of the burden. This makes it inappropriate to draw comparisons with the heroic and often constructive reaction to major disability which does not involve mental functions, such as spinal paralysis from trauma. Different again are patients who are mentally intact but who survive with physical diability, discomfort or pain and who are suffering from progressive disease. Sometimes these patients' problems are added to by side-effects and hazards of continuing treatment. Fortunately, there is now a greater willingness to consider quality and duration of survival in relation to treatment, which may be judged inadvisable quite apart from considerations of financial cost. What constitutes an acceptable quality of life is clearly a personal judgement; factors to consider are freedom from pain, ability to feed, dress and attend to personal toilet, capacity to organize daily life, to be mobile in the house and outside, to undertake social and leisure activities, and to work; both present satisfaction and future prospects affect the qualify of life.

Economics of Rescue

It has been stated that one of the main reasons for the escalating costs of medical care is that doctors now have the capacity to cure many more conditions than previously. Whilst most societies would want to try to meet the costs of treatment which has a high probability of resulting in cure, what concerns health economists is the enormous expense of treatment which is not in fact successful. Calculations of the actual costs are most readily available from North America, where item of service accounting is still customary. Cullen and his colleagues (8) reviewed costs for 226 critically ill postoperative patients and found that 21 per cent of the hospitalization charges (exclusive of physician's fees) went on blood products: 83 per cent of blood costs were expended on the 164 non-survivors. Both the blood costs and the overall charge per day were twice as great for fatal cases as for those who made full recovery.

The other side of the balance sheet is the cost of death – which rescue aims to avert. Aside from distress to relatives, which cannot be measured, this is usually calculated on the basis of years of lost livelihood. Awards by courts of law on this basis show all too clearly that all lives are not equal by this yardstick. Age is a critical determinant, in particular at the two ends of life. Under the age of 18 and over the age of 65 people are deemed to be unproductive, and death is therefore not considered to be associated with any loss of earning capacity; this might seem to be an unjust attitude to the potential of a talented young man nearly 18 years old. Yet the lives of many young and old persons are clearly valuable, not only to those around them but to society. Sometimes rescue can effectively reduce a state of continuing disability associated with inability to work or even of dependence – the clearest example is renal transplanation for a working man or the mother of a young family. In that case the equation is different, but the expected duration of survival after rescue must also be taken into account. Rescue after brain damage from head injury or after cardiorespiratory arrest, in a previously healthy individual, may result in prolonged survival with some degree of irrecoverable brain damage. In this case rescue has produced severe disability as a result of its 'success' in averting death – and the highest awards by courts for personal damages go to such patients. It is difficult to escape the view that this must be accounted an additional cost of rescue.

Another aspect of the cost of rescue for some patients is the benefit denied to other patients. There may be others in need of rescue procedures but with a better chance of making a reasonable recovery than those being treated – because such patients are apt to be the most critically ill, too often the hopelessly ill. But rescue procedures may also displace other more cost-effective activities, such as elective surgery for curable conditions. This is particularly apt to happen where facilities are common to both, and are stretched to capacity (3). Anaesthetists may spend a disproportionate amount of time in the intensive care unit, and consequently elective operation lists have to be curtailed; or an undue number of beds may be devoted to patients being rescued, or surviving after rescue. It is easier to delay the cure of patients on a surgical waiting list than to deny rescue to patients already in hospital, or presenting as emergency admissions. Consequently, many patients in surgical wards, when resources are restricted, are essentially incurable; meanwhile there are patients with curable conditions enduring months or years of suffering, disability and loss of work while they wait their turn to be cured.

Patient Selection

Most doctors dealing with rescue will acknowledge the immediate or ultimate futility of what they are doing for some of their patients. They continue to treat these patients because of demands made on them to do so, more often from other doctors than directly from patients and their relatives. Request for rescue may entail transfer of responsibility for a difficult problem to the rescue team, and the demands and the expectations of doctors referring such patients may be unrealistic and conflicting. Those involved in rescue may feel a need to accept cases or to continue treatment against their better judgement, because they are uncertain of support for a more rational approach; juniors may fear criticism from their seniors if they have not done 'everything', whilst those in one discipline may be concerned about criticism from another. In Britain it is unlikely that fear of legal redress figures largely in acute decision-making in this area, but it undoubtedly operates in North America. Clearly there is need for more open discussion about the selection of patients for initial rescue and also for the continuation of life-support.

Sometimes it is possible to involve several experts in a group discussion, such as selecting patients for renal transplantation, or for open heart surgery or for closure of severe spina bifida. More often the response to a request for rescue must be made rapidly. To help individual doctors in this position there is need for prior agreement about the principles which should be applied in selecting patients. Although there is less urgency about the decision to withdraw support, this difficult problem is also more easily solved if there have been prior discussions about principles. Skillman (12) has emphasized the importance of being prepared to discontinue treatment, and comments that evasion of this responsibility can produce serious deterioration in the morale of personnel in rescue teams, especially in intensive care units. There is no longer any serious argument against the withdrawal of support once patients are declared brain dead, but Skillman specifically states that a decision to discontinue treatment must often be made in less extreme or obvious circumstances. Decisions about admission and discharge should, he says, be based on consideration of the relative chances of survival of different patients; however, the likelihood of reasonable recovery should also be assured, because survival with severe disability may now be judged worse than death.

Whilst few would disagree with these principles, the lack of generally available predictive criteria about many of the conditions requiring rescue leaves many clinicians feeling that they have to treat all patients as though they had potential for recovery. There is urgent need, therefore, for the careful collection of data about patients with conditions requiring rescue, both so that predictions can be made in individual patients, and also to enable comparison of alternative treatment methods in formal trials on groups of patients. This requires standardization of methods of assessment of the initial severity and of the ultimate outcome. This represents a major undertaking but once a data bank has been collected it can be invaluable; Fries (13) claims that this may even make it possible to conduct therapeutic trials without a 'no treatment' group. When dealing with conditions associated with a high mortality it can be difficult to justify withholding even an unproven treatment from one group of patients, and comparison with a data bank could be particularly valuable in such circumstances.

Such data banks have been accumulated for patients with severe head injury (14) and for those with non-traumatic coma (15). The methods used in these two projects have been tested in several centres in different countries, and predictive criteria have emerged which enable a confident prediction to be made in almost half the patients during the first 24 hours of coma; the proportion which can be predicted increases as time passes during the first week. If triage is to be applied to candidates for rescue procedures then it should be based on firm data of this kind rather than on intuition or on unproven assumptions. However, Fried (16) claims that a doctor should not himself attempt to redistribute resources by withholding treatment from certain patients. He argues that triage is appropriate only in emergency situations – but it would seem reasonable to consider candidates for rescue as being in such a state. On the other hand, Skillman (12) maintains that lack of decision regarding triage is in effect a decision for the exclusion of those who need care but who cannot receive it, because they are not admitted to treatment.

A consensus on the principles which should apply to rescue triage should be reached not only amongst doctors in one clinical team or discipline, but should also involve other doctors, as well as health administrators and others whose task it is to monitor hospital activities. Unless there is agreement about such principles, individual doctors may not have the courage to take the rational rather than the traditional decision when faced with a rescue situation. It could even be that there would be a reluctance to embark on initial resuscitation because of the anticipated difficulty of discontinuing it, and this could begin to operate adversely even against patients who have a reasonable chance of making a good recovery after rescue.

Conclusions

Rescue procedures have become routine in acute hospitals in advanced Western countries. Unless there is a policy to guide patient selection, both for the initiation and for the withdrawal of rescue, then a disproportionate amount of resources are apt to be expended on such procedures – particularly in certain specialties or units. Unthinking application of rescue is disadvantageous not only to those patients whose treatment is denied or delayed because their need appears to be less pressing, but also to some of those who are rescued. More attention should be paid to the balance of benefits as well as of costs before patients with essentially incurable conditions are submitted to hazardous, unpleasant and elaborate treatment. This should include assessment of the probability of both short-term and long-term survival, and the quality of life which can reasonably be expected for survivors. Rationing of rescue is essential not only for the welfare of individual patients but also in order that the best use is made of the resources available for acute medical care. Hiatt (17) has drawn an analogy with herdsmen grazing on common land – once capacity is approached on the shared pasture, the attempts of individual herdsmen to increase their holdings has little benefit on the general welfare. Eventually, freedom on the commons brings ruin to all.

References

1. Hart, J.T. (1976). *Lancet,* ii, 731.
2. Maxwell, R. (1975). *British Medical Journal,* 3, 424.
3. Jennett, B. (1976). The way ahead for acute hospital services: delay cure, or deny rescue? *Lancet,* ii, 1235-1237.
4. Working Party (1975). Ethics of selective treatment of spina bifida. *Lancet,* i, 84.

5. Jennett, B. (1976). Resource allocation for the severely brain damaged. *Archives of Neurology,* **33,** 595.
6. Jennett, B., Teasdale, G., Galbraith, S., Pickard, J., Grant, H., Braakman, R., Avezaat, C., Maas, A., Minderhoud, J., Vecht, C.J., Heiden, J., Small, R., Caten, W. and Kurze, T. (1977). Severe head injuries in three countries. *Journal of Neurology, Neurosurgery and Psychiatry,* **40,** 291-298.
7. Caronna, J.J., Leigh, J., Shaw, D., Cartlidge, N., Knill-Jones, R. and Plum, F. (1975). The outcome of medical coma: prediction by bedside assessment of physical signs. *Transactions of the American Neurological Association,* **100,** 25.
8. Cullen, D.J., Ferrara, L.C., Briggs, B.A., Walker, P.F. and Gilbert, J. (1976). Survival, hospitalization charges and follow-up results in initially ill patients. *New England Journal of Medicine,* **294,** 982.
9. Bond, M. (1975). Assessment of the psychosocial outcome of severe head injury. In *Outcome of Severe Damage to the Central Nervous System,* Ciba Foundation Symposium 34, p. 141. Amsterdam, Excerpta Medica; London, Elsevier.
10. Jennett, B. and Bond, M. (1975). Assessment of outcome after severe brain damage. A practical scale. *Lancet,* i, 480.
11. Jennett, B. and Plum, F. (1972). Persistent vegetative state after brain damage. *Lancet,* i, 734.
12. Skillman, J.J. (1974). Ethical dilemmas in the care of the critically ill. *Lancet,* ii, 634.
13. Fries, J.F. (1976). A data bank for the clinician? *New England Journal of Medicine,* **294,** 1400.
14. Jennett, B., Teasdale, G., Braakman, R., Minderhoud, J. and Knill-Jones, R.P. (1976). Predicting outcome in individual patients after severe head injury. *Lancet,* i, 1031.
15. Caronna, J.J., Leigh, J., Shaw, D., Cartlidge, N., Knill-Jones, R. and Plum F. (1975). The outcome of medical coma: prediction by bedside assessment of physical signs. *Transactions of the American Neurological Association,* **100,** 25.
16. Fried, C. (1975). Rights and health care – beyond equity and efficiency. *New England Journal of Medicine,* **293,** 241.
17. Hiatt, H.H. (1975). Protecting the medical commons: who is responsible? *New England Journal of Medicine,* **293,** 235.

6

The Growth of Clinical Chemistry

L.G. Whitby

Many diseases have an underlying biochemical basis, and many other diseases give rise to metabolic disturbances. As knowledge of the biochemistry of disease has grown, so have the calls for chemical measurements to assist in the detection, diagnosis and treatment of disease.

The present pattern of requesting chemical measurements has built up over the last 30 years, following the development of inexpensive and reliable photoelectric colorimeters and flame photometers. To begin with, requests for investigation were almost entirely limited to those of a discretionary nature, defined as tests carried out in order to answer specific questions relating to the diagnosis of disease, or to assist with problems encountered in the management of illness. In the 1950s, although laboratories became very labour-intensive, the growing frequency of requests for chemical investigations was placing these departments under strain, as there were limits to the amount of additional space and staff that could be provided so as to handle the growing work-loads.

It is against this background of growing strain, inseparable from the maintenance of a reliable analytical service based on the repeated manual performance of techniques that were often complex and demanding, under precisely defined conditions, that the contribution of Skeggs should be seen. In 1957, Skeggs (1) described the first single-channel automatic chemical analyser, an instrument based on the principle of continuous flow analysis, in which specimens enter the system one after the other and the various chemical procedures, product detection and signal readout stages are carried out automatically on each specimen under closely controlled conditions.

The earliest continuous flow automatic analyser was designed as a versatile instrument. It soon proved to be both acceptable and amenable to development, and Table 6.1 summarizes the main stages through which developments have passed. The sequential multiple analysis plus computer

(SMAC) system, a multichannel analyser capable of performing up to 20 different chemical analyses on each specimen, includes as an essential component its own dedicated process-control computer.

Table 6.1
Developments in continuous flow analysers
(equipment manufactured by Technicon Instruments Corporation, Tarrytown, New York)

	Channels	*Chemistries available*	*Rate of analysis (specimens/hour)*	*Sample volume (ml)*	*Cost (£000)*	*Replacement cost (£000) (Sept. 1976)*
1957	1 (AAI)	+	20	2	2	5 (AAI)
1960	1 (AAI)	+	40	2	2	5 (AAI)
1962	1 (AAI)	+	60	2	2	5 (AAI), 6 (AAII)
1962	4 (AAI)	4	40	2	4 (AAI)	12(AAI),15(AAII)
1966	12(12/30)	12	30	2	20	Not available
1968	12(12/60)	12	60	2	24	65
1969	6 (6/60)	6	60	0.6	12	35
1971	12(SMA 12 Micro)	12	20	0.3	33	Not available
1973	4-12 (SMA Plus)	20	60	2	20-44	30-65
1974	20(SMAC)	23	150	0.4	114	133
1976	8(Micro-lyzer)	8	72	0.1	50	50

+Approximately 50 different chemical measurements have been satisfactorily adapted for performance on single-channel AutoAnalyzer I (AAI) equipment and these have since mostly been adapted for performance on single-channel AutoAnalyzer II (AAII) equipment, introduced in 1971 as an improvement upon AAI equipment.
SMA = simultaneous multiple analysis system
SMAC = sequential multiple analysis plus computer
Not available = no longer marketed

Clinical chemistry departments have become very dependent upon automatic analysers, of which continuous flow systems at present are the systems most commonly used. Several other automatic analysis systems (single-channel and multichannel) have been developed, in general based on different operating principles from continuous flow, and many of these other systems have come into service use in the last 5-10 years. The other important technical development in clinical chemistry has been the widespread introduction of computer-assisted process-control and data-processing systems, the largely numerical nature of chemical investigations facilitating the application of computers to this aspect of medical work. Much of this equipment is very expensive (Table 6.1) to purchase and to run, and it is often impossible to offset equipment costs by corresponding savings on staff salaries.

Automatic Analysers and Computers

One early consequence of introducing automatic analysers was to reduce the strain hitherto inseparable from the repetitive performance of much of the work of clinical chemistry laboratories, and this was accompanied by evidence of improved reliability of the results. More recently, the reduction in manual transcription consequent upon the introduction of computers into laboratories has further helped to improve standards of performance. These improvements have been bought at the cost of major capital expenditure.

Laboratories equipped with automatic analysers have a much greater capacity for analytical work, expressed on the basis of the average number of determinations performed by each technician, than departments where manual techniques predominate (Table 6.2), and the addition of computer technology has in some instances increased this analytical capacity still further. By removing at least temporarily the element of strain felt by

Table 6.2
Data for work-load, technical staff and automatic analysers
(Department of Clinical Chemistry, Royal Infirmary, Edinburgh)

Year	*Determinations*	*Specimens*	*Technical staff*	*Single-channel*	*Multichannel A*
1950	22,000	10,800	11	–	–
1955	57,000	36,400	14	–	–
1960	106,000	72,500	18	1	–
1963	195,000	95,800	23	3	–
1966	407,000	105,300	30	7	1 (5)
1969B	581,000	183,000	35	12	1 (5)
1972	779,000	246,000	40	14	1 (5)
1976	790,000 C	223,000 D	31	6	1 (14) E

A. The number of analytical channels on the multichannel analyser is shown in brackets.
B. A process-control computer has been used since 1969.
C. In 1974, chloride analyses (previously 98,000 p.a.) were discontinued.
D. Work from some hospitals has been transferred to another laboratory since 1972.
E. A 20-channel analyser, of which 14 channels were in service use in 1976 (16 in 1977).

laboratory staff when carrying out manual work on a large scale, the introduction of automatic analysers and computers has led to much greater use being made of chemical investigations, as could have been predicted by the application of Parkinson's law (2) which states that 'Work expands so as to fill the time available for its completion'. An example of expanding work-loads is given by the data contained in Table 6.2, for a laboratory that is still carrying out work mainly in response to requests of a purely discretionary nature (p. 56).

Another important consequence of the widespread adoption of automatic analysers, especially in laboratories operating fixed configuration multichannel systems, has been the alteration of internal laboratory organization so as to carry out a standard pattern of several tests, or 'profile of investigations', upon every specimen for which one or more of the tests included in the profile had been requested on a discretionary basis. Simplifying the internal organization of the laboratory's operations by standardizing the flow of work for many of the most frequently requested investigations is in itself an advantage to laboratory staff, but an additional advantage of test profiles is claimed to lie in the extra diagnostic information unexpectedly revealed by the performance of the standard profile of investigations, when compared with the amount of information gained from performing tests solely in response to discretionary requests (3) (Table 6.3). Profiles of investigations, especially when all

Table 6.3
Comparison of routine laboratory findings and admission profiles

	Routine laboratory	*Profile laboratory*
Total patients having chemical investigations	477	623
Total determinations	2,206	6,853
Total abnormalities found	191	340
Patients with abnormalities	120	226

Distribution of the 149 additional abnormalies revealed by the profile investigations:

	Total	*'Medically significant'*
Sugar	31	16
Urea	7	4
Sodium	10	0
Potassium	25	1
Chloride	2	0
Total carbon dioxide	6	1
Calcium	6	1
Phosphorus	10	2
Protein	15	2
Albumin	9	4
Urate	28	23

Data from Bryan et al. (3).

results are reported whether or not the tests have been requested, have contributed greatly to the increase (self-generated) in work in many clinical chemistry laboratories.

Another consequence of the development of high capacity automatic analysers, and computer-assisted data processing, has been the growing range of laboratory measurements in screening programmes of the apparently healthy population, or in health check-ups on selected groups of people. Many multiphasic screening or regular health check programmes are now in operation in the United States, and these mostly incorporate a large number of clinical chemistry and haematology tests.

The Growth of Clinical Chemistry: is it all Worthwhile?

Data collected by the Health Departments and by the Office of Health Economics show that, in the last 10-20 years, the growth in use of diag-

Table 6.4
Profiles of chemical investigations

(The performance of a standard range of measurements whenever one or more of the tests included in the range is requested on a discretionary basis)

ADVANTAGES

1. *To the clinician*
   (a) The earlier detection, in a small proportion of patients, of information leading to more precise diagnosis, or an important change in diagnosis, and hence to the possible earlier institution of more appropriate treatment.
   (b) The automatic performance of a range of chemical measurements early in the course of patients' illnesses (data not necessarily all immediately reported), with associated greater opportunities for monitoring the progress of disease.
   (c) Simplification of requesting procedures where profiles of investigations become one of the standard options available to clinicians.
2. *To the laboratory*
   (a) Standardized pattern of work-flow for some of the most frequently requested investigations, with associated savings on staff costs or opportunities for staff redeployment for the performance of tests for which there is hitherto unmet clinical demand.

DISADVANTAGES

1. *To the clinician*
   (a) Where results of unrequested investigations are reported, annoyance caused if the amount of unrequested data causes difficulty in comprehension (data flood).
   (b) Where profiles are offered as a standard option, reduction in the need to consider why some tests might be needed, with consequent loss of critical approach to the requesting of laboratory investigations.
2. *To the laboratory*
   (a) Possible increased dependence on high level technology (e.g. for operating multichannel analysers and computer systems), and consequent greater dependence on manufacturers' service organizations.
   (b) Greater service operating costs in terms of expenditure on chemicals, etc., as compared with the equivalent needs for discretionary analysis.

NOTES

1. Although stated in somewhat categorical terms, these advantages and disadvantages should only be regarded as generalizations, and subject to considerable local modification.
2. Many of these statements are only amenable to value judgements about their effectiveness and any benefits or defects; precise cost-benefit analysis is not applicable.

nostic services provided by laboratory departments has been associated with some of the greatest percentage increases in calls made upon health care resources. At a time of financial stringency, it is natural to ask whether the growing dependence of doctors upon laboratory investigations is fully justified, or alternatively whether all the extra tests performed nowadays (as compared with 20 years ago) are worthwhile. It is easy to point to the increasing costs of diagnostic services, but it is much more difficult to relate these increasing costs unequivocally to improvements in patient care or to the prevention of illness.

One aspect of clinical chemistry work which has come under particular scrutiny has been the justification for profile investigations, and Table 6.4 attempts to summarize the principal advantages and disadvantages of this relatively recent change in laboratory practice. The criticisms seem mainly to stem from two propositions:

1. When profile investigations are reported that were not requested on a discretionary basis, the fact that extra work has been performed must necessarily imply additional expense in the provision of the laboratory service.
2. Where doctors have become accustomed to laboratories performing standard profiles of laboratory investigations, this has reduced the critical element in the selection of appropriate tests and has not improved standards of diagnosis. Indeed, the flood of data automatically generated by multichannel analysers is thought by some to have impeded the decision-making process.

As far as the first of these criticisms is concerned, it is important to stress that the operation of a standard pattern of single-channel automatic analysers, or the equivalent multichannel analyser(s), for the regular performance of a profile of investigations has been shown to be relatively economical in terms of the numbers of staff required to operate the equipment, as compared with the numbers required to perform the identical range of investigations but solely on a discretionary basis. Although it might appear to be wasteful of reagents, to the extent that these are used in the performance of some unrequested investigations, in general the extra expenditure on reagents is more than offset by the staff savings. Whether or not to report the results of profile investigations, other than those speciifically requested, is a matter for local decision, a decision which needs to take account of the ethical consequences of failing to report data for unrequested examinations even though the results may suggest the presence of an unsuspected abnormality. Where unrequested data have been reported, by laboratories performing standard profiles of investigations, it is unfortunately true that the additional yield of diagnostic information has been low (4), and unexplained abnormal findings have led to extra work (5). This last fact has led to some outspoken condemnations of admission profile (sometimes called screening) methods of investigation (6).

It is more difficult to comment on the second set of criticisms. By reducing the element of choice in the selection of tests, the performance and regular reporting of profiles of investigations can cause difficulties in interpretation of data. This is because the relative non-specificity of many chemical measurements means that, for the proper understanding of each set of data, there should have been a reason for requesting each investigation (7). Even more unfortunate has been the experience of some laboratories that the regular reporting of large numbers of results (e.g. 20 sets of chemical investigations on every patient when first admitted to hospital) has led to instances where important information has been overlooked, or the ability to comprehend so much data at one time has been inadequate. To some extent these pitfalls have been overcome by the use of computer-assisted report preparation (p. 65).

There is, in fact, no simple answer to the question whether the growth of clinical chemistry has been worthwhile – the answer is related to the viewpoint of the questioner. Much of the growth has been made possible by expenditure on automatic analysers and computers, but it is reasonable to question whether, in every case, the right tests have been made more readily available by automation. What the automatic analysers have achieved is the easier performance, on a large scale, of the tests that were hitherto being requested and performed manually in large numbers, but these are not necessarily the best tests for helping doctors with problems in diagnosis. Few would question the statement that investment in automation has enabled clinical chemistry laboratories to meet the increasing calls made upon the diagnostic services they offer, although this is begging the question as to whether these calls (which are responsible for the continuing growth in usage) are in themselves worthwhile, or to what extent they represent wasteful use of resources.

What Might be Done to Give Better Value for Money?

Education. There have been many pronouncements, mostly imperfectly substantiated, about the extent to which laboratory services are over-used, misused, or even frankly abused. Criticisms about over-use sometimes relate to the requesting of repeated sets of investigations at intervals which are too short in relation to the rate of development of the disease process (e.g. the requesting of a range of liver function tests on a daily basis), or the unselective requesting of every investigation that might be, in greater or lesser degree, contributory (e.g. the routine measurement of several enzyme activities in all patients suspected of having had a myocardial infarction, regardless of the interval between the onset of the illness and the time of collecting the blood samples; or the routine performance of the same six or more chemical tests of thyroid function without first considering which are particularly appropriate for investigating suspected hypothyroidism, as distinct from suspected hyperthyroidism). Other criticisms suggesting over-use or misuse of laboratory services have been more directed at the laboratories themselves, in relation to the reporting of unrequested work as part of a set of profile investigations (6).

Theoretically, laboratories might overcome criticisms relating to over-use of their facilities, as a component of unjustifiable growth, by introducing a system requiring adequate justification by clinical staff of every request for chemical investigations, coupled with a strictly discretionary system of reporting work. Such a system would almost invariably fail in practice, because clinical chemistry is one of the shortage specialties in medical practice and, even if there were to be adequate numbers of medically qualified clinical chemists, it is still difficult for laboratory-based staff to question the clinical justification for laboratory investigations without giving rise to adverse reactions. A few laboratories include, as part-time members of their staff, doctors who are primarily practising as clinicians, and some medically qualified clinical chemists regularly practise as part-time clinicians, but usually only in limited fields of medical practice; neither of these somewhat exceptional arrangements can be expected to contribute greatly to reducing problems of over-use or misuse of laboratory investigations, and most heads of laboratories have found, in practice, that it is better to organize their service so as to meet demand.

There is, nevertheless, one general approach that might help to solve the problems presented by over-use or misuse of chemical investigations, this approach requiring a reassessment of priorities in undergraduate medical education. At the postgraduate level, it has for several years been recognized that it is no longer appropriate to think in terms of hospital pathology departments, since specialization (and indeed subspecialization) within pathology has become the established pattern for a modern laboratory service. The growing diversification of laboratory medicine is being increasingly reflected in the pattern of its organization into separate departments of clinical chemistry, haematology and blood transfusion, microbiology, morbid anatomy and histopathology, and into inter-disciplinary subjects such as immunology. Specialization within laboratory medicine ('pathology') is recognized in programmes of postgraduate education and in the related specialized diploma examinations, as well as in the changing pattern of specialist appointments. The same cannot be said, as yet, for the education of undergraduate medical students since, in most medical schools, teaching about the pathological basis of disease is still mainly the preserve of histopathologists and microbiologists. There is insufficient recognition of the growing importance of biochemical disturbances as causes of disease, or as important factors contributing to complications, and the young discipline of clinical chemistry usually receives a relatively minute allocation of time in the undergraduate curriculum. Until this situation is remedied, it is likely that doctors will continue to qualify to practise medicine while possessing an inadequate awareness of the value and limitations of clinical chemistry in diagnosis and management of illness.

Cut Back on the Present Facilities. For this course of action to be justified, it is necessary for its proponents to specify what facilities should be curtailed. It is true that some clinical chemistry laboratories continue to perform outdated tests, but it is even more true that most laboratories are justifiably under pressure to extend the range of investigations they can offer to clinicians. It is also fair to suggest that, while many doctors could probably continue to practise reasonable standards of medicine with a severely curtailed range of chemistry services, few would wish to be denied access to laboratory facilities to the extent required to make major financial savings. The main areas of growth in clinical chemistry, as measured in terms of numbers of investigations performed, have been in the relatively simple, inexpensive, frequently requested and easily automated investigations, and the more expensive methods of investigation are mostly to be found among measurements which have only become available in the last 5-10 years (e.g. many isoenzyme, specific protein and hormone measurements). To a large extent, the ability of chemistry laboratories to introduce some of these recent tests has depended on the existence of automatic analysers and computers for carrying out the major load of repetitive analytical work. To cut back on existing levels of investment, in staff or equipment, could severely limit the possibilities for improving the specificity of chemical diagnosis that would follow from the wider use of new, specialized and sometimes technically very demanding measurements.

Rationalize the Provision of Clinical Chemistry Laboratories. There is increasing specialization within clinical chemistry, as one consequence of growing understanding of the biochemical basis of disease. However, at the same time, clinical chemistry is one of the shortage specialties. There is, therefore, a case for concentrating scarce expertise into a relatively small number of large laboratories serving large sections of the population, rather than continue to provide large numbers of relatively small laboratories each attempting to offer a reasonable range of modern diagnostic services. Rationalization of services is also relevant to any attempt to derive maximum utilization in return for major capital investment in high capacity multichannel analysers such as the Technicon SMAC system (Table 6.1) and in computer-assisted data-processing systems for report generation and records storage.

Rationalization of laboratory services is a complex subject. It is not always easy to plan clinically acceptable provision of the laboratory services for a population, or a group of hospitals, around one major laboratory (with its associated capacity for handling large work-loads) and related satellite laboratories. Every situation where rationalization might be contemplated demands careful study, and the interests of patients and the reasonable requirements of clinicians have to be balanced against the feasibility of staffing and financing the various forms of laboratory service which might be provided.

Computer-assisted Reporting of Data. Assuming that the present level of use of chemical investigations is likely to continue, or even to continue to grow, some of the problems associated with the assimilation by clinicians of the data contained in laboratory reports merit brief consideration.

It can be argued that it is wasteful to carry out a range of chemical measurements (e.g. as part of a profile of investigations) and then discard all except the results for those tests requested on a discretionary basis. Computer-assisted data processing, however, offers the possibility of storing all the data and reporting selectively. For instance, selective reporting could be restricted to the reporting of discretionary tests, or extended to include the results of discretionary tests and those additional investigations included in the profile for which the unrequested findings proved to be markedly abnormal. Non-reported data would, in either case, be available for recall if required, and could be consulted retrospectively, assuming that doctors were made aware that such extra information could be made available if found to be potentially relevant.

Other ways in which computer-assisted reporting of data have begun to assist doctors in comprehending the 'flood' of figures emerging from clinical chemistry laboratories include the automatic flagging of results which are so abnormal as to demand explanation, the expression of all results in terms of the number of standard deviations by which they differ from the mean for the healthy population, and computer-assisted interpretation of groups of related investigations. Diagnosis by computer, based on the results of chemical measurements alone, is still a long way from attainment, but computer-assisted interpretation of liver function tests, thyroid function tests and acid-base balance data provide three examples of ways in which some laboratories now amplify their hitherto predominantly numerical reports, the laboratory data sometimes being coupled in this computer analysis with appropriate clinical information.

Conclusion

The growth of clinical chemistry stems partly from the growing understanding of the biochemical basis of disease, which has led to a requirement for the introduction of new methods of diagnosis based on chemical measurements. It has also resulted from the increasingly frequent use made by doctors of chemical investigations of a long-established nature, on a discretionary requesting basis, and from the decision of many laboratories to organize the handling of some components of their rising work-loads on a simplified work-flow or standardized basis, resulting in the introduction of profiles of investigations.

Responsible utilization of laboratory services demands better education of doctors. It is not considered appropriate to restrict the use of chemical investigations by means of arbitrary curbs, although comparisons between costings in different laboratories might reveal examples of wasteful use of resources. Information bearing on this subject has begun to be collected by the Health Departments and by the Royal College of Pathologists, in their compilation of data relating to laboratory staffing, patterns of work-load and major items of equipment.

References

1. Skeggs, L.T. (1957). *American Journal of Clinical Pathology,* 28, 311.
2. Parkinson, C.N. (1958). *Parkinson's Law.* London, John Murray.
3. Bryan, D.J., Wearne, J.L., Viau, A., Musser, A.W., Schoonmaker, F.W. and Thiers, R.E. (1966). *Clinical Chemistry,* 12, 137.
4. Whitehead, T.P. and Wootton, I.D.P. (1974). *Lancet,* ii, 1439.
5. Durbridge, T.C., Edwards, F., Edwards, R.G. and Atkinson, M. (1976). *Medical Journal of Australia,* 1, 703.
6. Rhodes, P. (1976). *British Medical Journal,* 2, 804.
7. Asher, R. (1954). *British Medical Journal,* 2, 460.

7

Implications of an Ageing Population

Sir John Brotherston and W.T. Thom

It was Bernard Barouch in 1951 who said that the increase of man's lifespan by 18 years in a period of 50 years was more revolutionary and had more profound medical, economic and social implications than such things as atomic energy, air transport and modern communications (1). The main factors responsible for most of this increase have been the reduction of infant and childhood mortality and the control of infection in midspan.

The elderly are increasing more rapidly than the total population, and this, combined with the reduction in working hours, has produced considerable changes in society.

This process of demographic change is predictable as it is based not on the imponderable forward estimates of birth rates but on people whose survival can be accurately calculated.

In Scotland the demographic changes during this century have shown a steep rise in the population over 65 years of age which continues until about 1980 when it begins to level off. The over-75-years group, however, continues to increase well into the 1990's. These very old people make some of the heaviest demands on the Health Service.

Figure 7.1 demonstrates the changes which have occurred and can be expected over the next 20 years in Scotland. While these show the national situation, there are great local variations. In 1974 the proportion of elderly in the population was as low as 9.5 per cent in Lanarkshire and as high as 18 per cent in the Western Islands.

The greater survival rate of women in Western society is another important factor in the equation. Widowed, divorced and single women form a high proportion of the patients in departments of geriatric medicine. Marriage would appear to have a strong protective effect and couples seem capable by mutual support to contrive to live longer in the community.

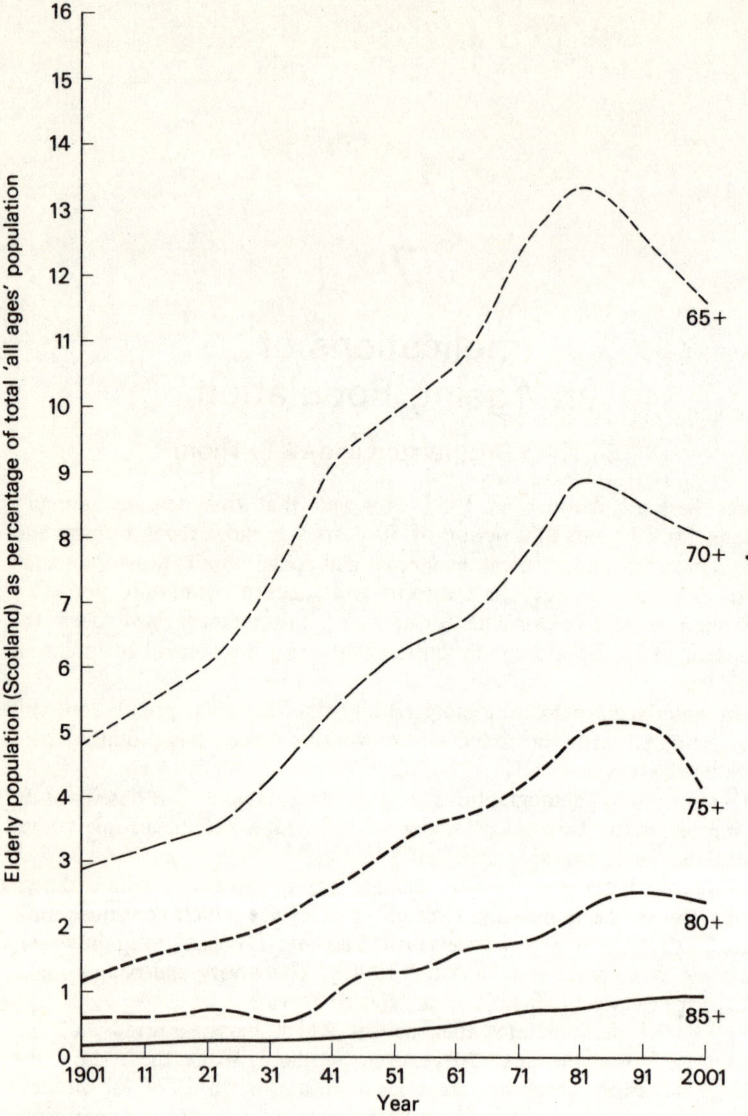

Figure 7.1.

Traditionally the middle-aged female has carried the main burden of supporting the elderly and the gradual decrease in this midspan population over the next 20 years is a factor of note which is demonstrated in Figs. 7.2.

There is little basis for the assertion that the family is failing to discharge its responsibilities towards the elderly. By far the biggest support

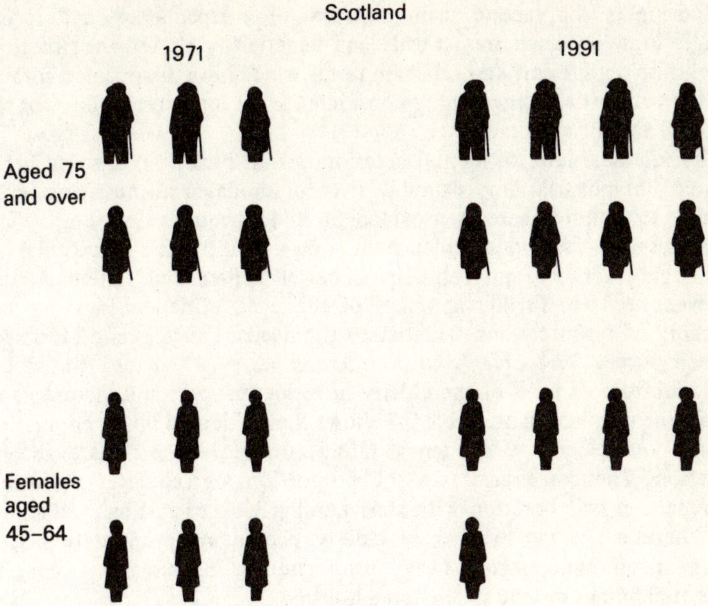

Figure 7.2.

service for the elderly in the community is the family – in its widest sense, including neighbours. Professor Isaacs' work in Glasgow showed that the outstanding cases of rejection to which more publicity is given are usually persons with a history of previous breakdown of family relationships due to actions of the elderly person in earlier life (2).

When a community with this kind of demographic scene is examined, what solutions are available for the care of the elderly? As stated by Peter Townsend (3), the first objective is to enlarge and preserve the individual's capacity for independence. Retention of personal identity and respect for the need for privacy are essential and the safeguard or restoration of health and the capacity to undertake personal and household activities are factors of great importance in the retention of independence.

The health professions, particularly, are prone to think of old age in terms of pathology and to forget that about 95 per cent of the elderly live independently, albeit with varying degrees of family and other support. There is, however, an elderly minority which, although a small percentage, still constitutes a large number of people whose demands create strain on our systems and resources.

Independence can be assisted by cash or by kind. Pensions in the UK still compare unfavourably with several other European countries. The tradition has been to provide service and facilities, but the simple income solution merits more consideration than in the past.

Housing is the second main platform of independence, and recent changes in policy have dramatically and beneficially altered the situation. 'Poorhouse' and 'eventide home' are terms which have disappeared forever and the residential home is now considered as a supportive facility for the very frail and incapacitated.

The tolerable level of mental deterioration in such homes is still being debated but physical illness should be accommodated in most cases even through to terminal care as provided in an individual's own home. The seriousness of lost independence is now realized and the value of encouraging activity and self-help is better appreciated. There is still, however, need for further appraisal of the levels of dependency and the matching of resources and facilities to the needs. Carstairs and Morrison, in their survey *The Elderly in Residential Care* (4), demonstrated the wide spectrum of need of the elderly in residential care and the problems of possible misplacement. Table 7.1 shows the residential home population assessed on selected dependency ratings for more appropriate accommodation. The percentages are the proportions agreed after individual assessment in collaboration with staff familiar with each subject. It shows that there is a large number of elderly people inappropriately placed taking up an unnecessarily heavy proportion of resources by being in residential homes instead of sheltered housing.

Table 7.1.
Survey of homes for the elderly: allocation of residents to most appropriate types of care

Number of residents assessed	10,906
Sheltered housing	29.6%
Residential home	50.8%
Home for mentally frail	7.2%
Hospital	12.4%

From Carstairs and Morrison (4).

Recent developments in the field of housing are of great importance and could be moving in the proper direction for a solution to this problem.

Sheltered housing – small, well designed, grouped, housing connected to a warden service by an efficient communication system – provides facilities for the support of elderly people in partial independence. Different methods have been developed in different countries, but a recent policy initiative in Scotland has been to encourage local authorities and housing associations to provide sheltered housing or housing capable of easy conversion to the sheltered concept so that elderly people can be retained in their own familiar community.

Figure 7.3 shows diagrammatically the different forms of housing involved and suggests alternatives which can be made to change a complex to suit an area's changing needs (5). Such a complex provides the basic facilities on which a structure for the proper care of the elderly can be

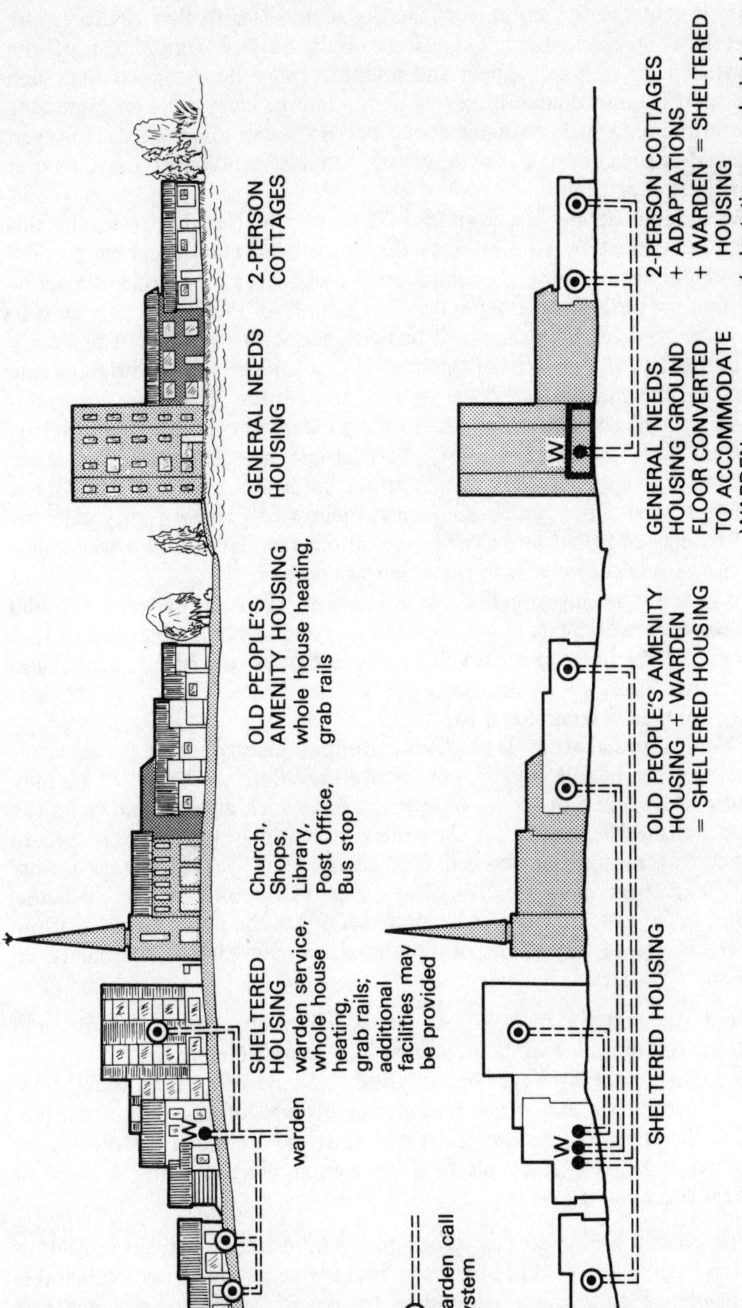

Figure 7.3 (Reproduced with permission of the Controller of HMSO (5i).)

built. It requires the support of the Social and Health Services to ensure maximum independence. The Home Help Service forms one of the essential parts of this support and present observations suggest that such services will require large increases if they are to carry the ever increasing responsibilities which changing social patterns heap upon them. However, financial stringency and scarcity of suitable candidates may restrict immediate expansion.

When considering the responsibilities of the Health Service in this situation it must be stressed that the majority of elderly people are just part of the normal general population for whom it is one aid, and a necessary one, in prolonging independence. The duty of the Health Service is to meet the need of the moment of this group as with any other. The elderly are entitled to the services of the general practitioner and the primary care team, or the hospital services, as the need arises. There are, however, certain special considerations due to the greater vulnerability of the ageing physique, the increased liability to multiple pathology and the lesser capacity for rapid recovery which affect the health needs of the elderly. The present stoicism which frequently delays or prevents early calls for services may not continue as new generations familiar with the availability and use of services move into the upper age groups.

As a result of investigations in Sweden in 1961, it was demonstrated that those over 80 years of age received two and one-half times the average amount of medical care provided. These figures are based on demand rather than need so are probably an underestimate. Figure 7.4 sets out these results in diagrammatic form.

Where a special study is made of a group of elderly people by a doctor, nurse or other health worker, commonly they find conditions which may or may not be known to the old person but which are not known to the medical authorities, including the general practitioner (6). There is need to look at the responsibilities and objectives of the Health Service against this background of morbidity. The needs, as opposed to the demands, require to be assessed. The philosophy set out in the notable report of the Royal College of Physicians of Edinburgh on the care of the elderly in Scotland (7) stated this clearly:

> First, the elderly must be supported in independence, comfort and contentment in their own homes for as long as possible.
>
> Secondly, alternative accommodation must be offered to those who, from infirmity or any other reason, are in need of care and attention.
>
> Thirdly, hospital accommodation must be provided promptly for those who, by reason of physical or mental ill-health, are in need of medical and nursing care.

The elderly are an at risk group in whom acute illness, surgical intervention, compulsory retirement or bereavement can erode vulnerable independence and whose reluctance to ask for services can complicate the problem.

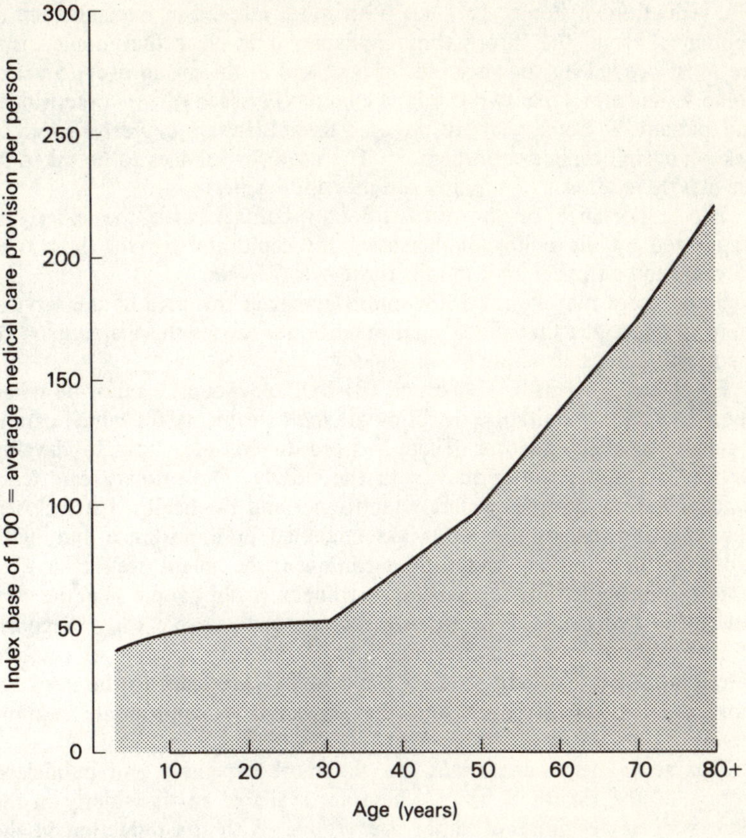

Figure 7.4 Medical care at different ages in Sweden (From Maxwell (7i).)

The first point of contact is usually with the general practitioner. It is a fact that the greatest volume of medical care for the elderly is provided by the general practitioner, in partnership with the District Nursing and Health Visitor Services and, in some cases, the social worker. In Scotland a policy of primary care provided from Health Centre bases has been adopted and an ambitious programme of Health Centre building is in progress. Health centres provide a focal point at which general practitioners and consultants in geriatric medicine can meet, where comprehensive services for the elderly (including consultant clinics) can be developed. The centralization of services at health centres can, however, produce problems of accessibility for the elderly with their reduced mobility. The work of Elliot and Stevenson (8) demonstrated how some recent developments in general practice may operate adversely for the elderly. The changing attitude to home visits is important to the older patients.

The reduction in home visits has been more marked in England than in Scotland. From the information available, it is clear that home visits are most needed by the very old. In Scotland in the group over 75 years, home visits form some two-thirds of contacts between general practitioner and patient. If home visits to the aged diminish there could be a serious risk of overall reduction in contact. The need for services to be taken to the elderly requires examination and new approaches.

The importance of the patient/doctor contact with the elderly is recognized by the policy of increasing the capitation fee for those over 65 years and a further addition for those over 75 years.

While there may be room for improvement in this area of the service, there is no doubt that the general practitioner carries the major share of the health burden in caring for the elderly.

Elliot and Stevenson also noted (8) that old people cannot be relied upon to take the initiative to bring all their problems for which care is required to their doctors. There is need to consider how to develop services, to ensure the contact with the elderly. The primary care team concept has brought the general practitioner and the health visitor closer. The contribution of the latter has increased in importance and, with additional training in diagnostic techniques, she might well take over more responsibility for supervision of vulnerable old people (e.g. the very old, those living alone, the recently bereaved) to enable early diagnosis of many conditions – depression, loss of mobility, cardiac or cerebral deterioration, etc. – and so alert the primary care team to the need for more detailed investigation and the provision of appropriate support services.

The acute hospital services are the most expensive and publicized section of the Health Services. These are available to the elderly in the same way as to those of other age groups. With the reduction in the volume of morbidity due to infection, degenerative disease processes constitute the major portion of the morbidity in hospital today. The degenerative diseases are more closely associated with advancing years and as a result the elderly population are the heaviest users of the hospital system. It must be accepted that the elderly will require practically every specialty and every department and that hospital medicine will more and more be concerned with the care of older patients. It is a fact that the majority of old people who enter hospital are admitted to acute beds. The geriatric departments have special responsibilities for assessment, rehabilitation and long-term care which requires a considerable number of beds.

The usage by the elderly of hospital beds in terms of admissions and of bed days occupied over the last decade has recently been computed in Scotland. Over the period 1962-1971 there was a reduction of occupied bed days by the midspan population, but this has been taken up by the elderly. Figure 7.5 shows the changes occuring over this period.

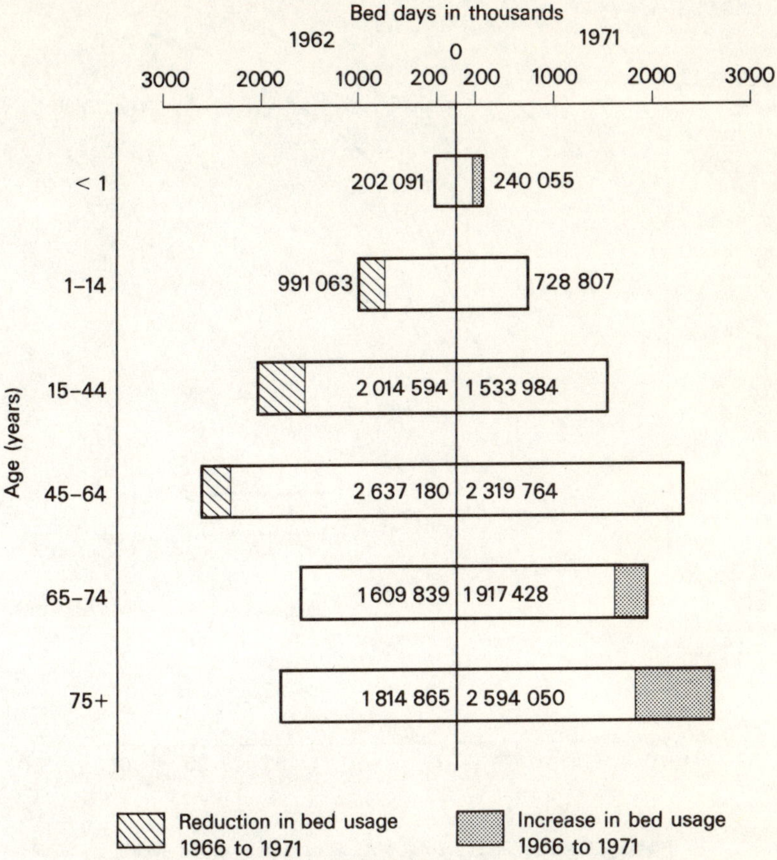

Figure 7.5 In-patient bed utilization comparison: 1962-1971. (Information Services Division, Common Service Agency)

When this increase is shown in linear form from 1960 and projected forwards to the end of the century, it shows a steady increase in the use of hospital beds by the elderly. This is a hypothetical situation but continuation of these present trends would require an increase of nearly 4,000 beds for the care of elderly by 1990 and this is demonstrated in Fig. 7.6.

If one looks at the discharges from non-psychiatric hospitals, it can be seen that the responsibility for caring for patients over 65 years of age is spread over all specialties. In Fig. 7.7 this is shown for the year 1974.

Not surprisingly, 90 per cent of those discharged from departments of geriatric medicine are over 65 years of age, but the proportion from general medicine and other specialties is also high and even such specialties as plastic surgery and neurosurgery are involved.

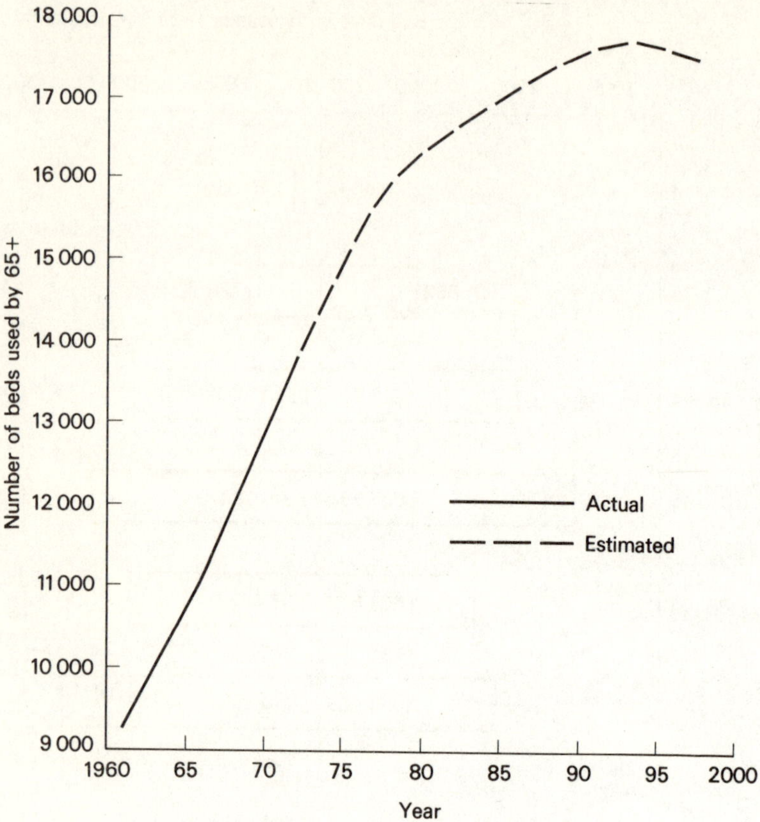

Figure 7.6 Actual and forecast of beds used daily, 1961-1998. (Information Services Division, Common Service Agency)

There is no doubt some measure of misplacement but it is difficult to isolate the cause and produce a solution. In one study by the Nuffield Hospitals Trust (9) 5 per cent of beds in teaching hospital medical units were found to be occupied by patients who would have been more appropriately placed in departments of geriatric medicine. This 5 per cent causes much argument and considerable misunderstanding but nevertheless they need appropriate care.

Forty-five per cent of the occupancy of all mental hospitals is by patients over 65 years of age and in the female wards it is over 50 per cent. This population is comprised partly of 'graduates', i.e. those who have grown old in hospitals, having been admitted in the past when long-term hospitalization was the accepted treatment for many psychiatric conditions. There is, however, a growing proportion of elderly first admissions, especially of patients who are dementing. This whole question of geriatric psychiatry constitutes a challenge and much debate continues in the

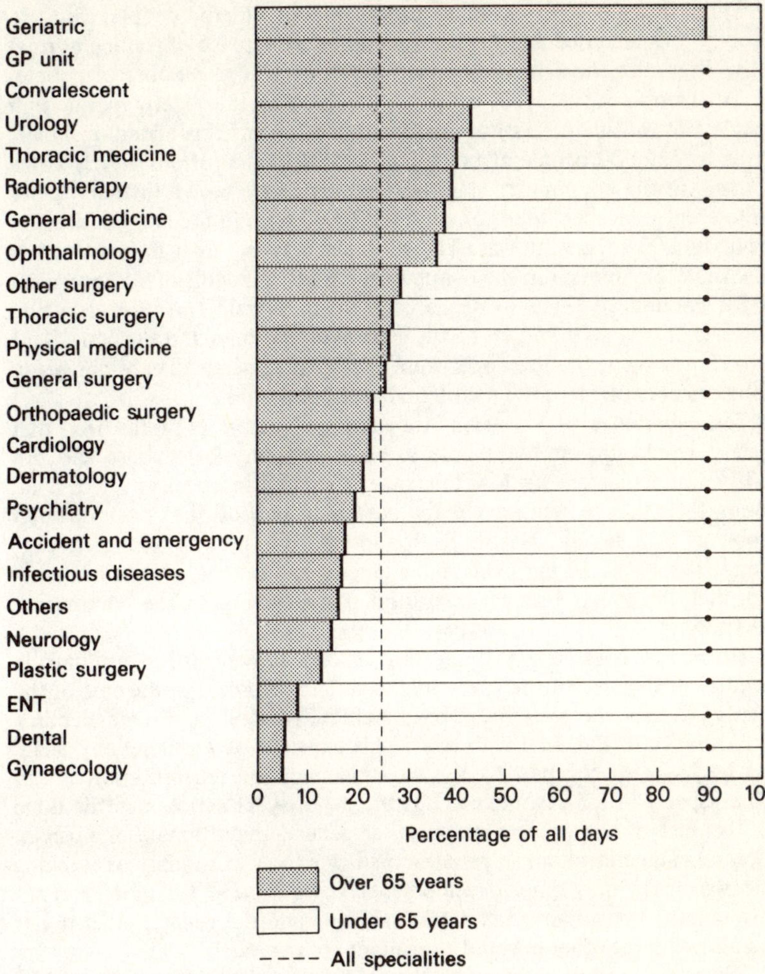

Figure 7.7 Discharges from Scottish non-psychiatric hospitals in 1974, by age and unit of discharge. (Information Services Division, Common Service Agency)

specialty of psychiatry on how these patients should be treated and by whom.

The geriatric day hospital is a comparatively recent development. The original concept was for rehabilitation, but in practice many patients attend for considerable periods. The availability of day centres for social support of the elderly affects the demands made on day hospitals. Transport is essential for such units and there are problems in its provision. Careful assessment of these different needs is necessary for the efficient provision of day hospital care.

While there is only a small proportion of elderly people who are severely incapacitated and the great majority are capable of leading normal active lives, this small fraction constitutes a very large number of people. In Townsend's survey (10) only 2.1 per cent of the elderly population (inside and outside of institutions) were bedfast but this added up in UK terms to 129,000 people at home and 77,000 in institutions, nearly twice as many in the community as in institutions. There were a further 4.2 per cent severely incapacitated, of whom 250,000 were in the community and about 84,000 in institutions. The problem may be great in hospital but how much greater is it in the community? What standards of care are given in the community? The evidence of incredible strain and utter devotion which is all too well known to the general practitioner and the consultant in geriatric medicine give one cause for great concern. There are many instances of caring in quite unacceptable circumstances.

The experience of Ferguson Anderson and others (11) has been that society would appear to be able to cope with physical disease and disability but it has a very low tolerance of mental incapacity. There is no doubt that the dementing elderly person is one of the most difficult problems in a family. Martin Roth and his colleagues in Newcastle (12) found that about 10 per cent of the elderly had some degree of dementia and that for every 1 in an institution there were 6 in the community situation.

There has been much discussion on the role of the consultant in geriatric medicine and the place of the geriatric services in the care of the elderly. Clearly the geriatrician has rehabilitative skills and understanding of morbidity in the elderly to add to his expertise as a general physician, and he has a special part to play in assessment and rehabilitation and in some aspects of long-term care. But the majority of caring must be done by the rest of the profession (whether general practitioners or hospital doctors). The consultant in geriatric medicine has a missionary or teaching role which requires more development. There is need for more contact between the consultant in geriatric medicine and the general practitioner and also with his other hospital consultant colleagues.

There is also need to examine the attitudes of the health professions – medicine, nursing, etc. There are still outdated attitudes that the laudable patient is one who is young and acutely ill who rapidly recovers or dies. The sense of grievance which develops when elderly patients in teaching wards are delayed in discharge because of loss of independence for one cause or another is irrational. The fault does not lie with the patient but with the need to find the right solution through the development of correct partnerships and professional interactions. Correct attitudes must be learnt from the environment in which medical and nursing students grow up.

The Health Service is only one of a number of services involved in making the right kind of environment for an ageing community and seeking the correct solution. Social Work Services and Housing are at least as important, and the great challenge is whether these service boundaries can be crossed and a joint solution found. There are no separate populations of 'health service' or 'social work' or 'housing' elderly. It is necessary to develop a total approach to provide for a spectrum of needs by a spectrum of services for one population of old people. The reorganization of the Health Services has set in motion, with the development of Programme Planning Groups (Area Health Care Planning Teams), joint activity in thinking in these terms, and, properly used and developed, could do much to find the correct solution.

While the statutory services can do much and the professionals have much to contribute, the main support must and does come from the community and the relatives of the elderly. Voluntary effort is a large and important part of the support and must be well guided and integrated into the whole structure of services. The work of Age Concern and other voluntary agencies in recruitment of helpers and training of personnel is extremely valuable. The importance of skilled guidance and education in the proper approach to the elderly must be stressed. Tactless interference with independence can do much harm. One of our greatest untapped sources of help is the younger elderly. The psychological benefit of positive action for them and the great value of their contribution toward the care and support of the older age groups is clear.

Should the physical provision for the geriatric service be less attractive than other parts of the system? The environment and the supporting services are important not only to the old people directly but also indirectly because of the morale of caring staff. In the long run may it be a better buy to invest in services for the elderly than to opt for some attractive addition at the acute end of the system which may benefit fewer patients?

Basic decisions on the use of Health Service resources are often made by the professionals. Doctors have great influence through their advisory systems and decisions on priorities are difficult to implement without the support of the medical and other staff. The UK is in a period of financial difficulty and the Health Service can expect little growth for some time after a long period of considerable expansion. During this latter period the most privileged part of the service has been the acute hospital service, Consideration should be given to allocating a greater share to longer term caring responsibilities; this would in turn relieve pressure on the acute services.

References

1. Leavell, H.R. and Clark, E.G. (1958). *Preventive Medicine for the doctor in his community: an epidemiological approach,* 2nd edn., p. 434. New York and Maidenhead, McGraw-Hill.
2. Isaacs, B. (1971). Studies of Illness and Death in the Elderly in Glasgow. Scottish Health Service Studies No 17. Scottish Home and Health Department.

3. Townsend, P. (1962). *The Last Refuge.* London, Routledge & Kegan Paul.
4. Carstairs, V. and Morrison, M. (1971). The Elderly in Residential Care. Scottish Health Service Studies No 19. Scottish Home and Health Department.
5. Scottish Development Department (1975). *Housing for the Elderly:* (i) SDD Circular No. 120/1975; (ii) SWSG Circular No. SW/25/1975. Edinburgh, HMSO.
6. Williamson, J., Stokoe, I.H., Gray, S., Fisher, M., Smith, A., McGhee, A. and Stephenson, E. (1964). Old people at home – their unreported needs. *Lancet,* i, 1117.
7. Royal College of Physicians, Edinburgh (1963). *The Care of the Elderly in Scotland.* Report of a Committee. Edinburgh, Royal College of Physicians.
7i. Maxwell, R.J. (1974). *Health Care: the growing dilemma.* New York and London, McKinsey & Co.
8. Elliot, A.E. and Stevenson, J.S.K. (1973). Geriatric care in general practice. *Journal of the Royal College of General Practitioners,* **23,** 615.
9. Meredith, J., Anderson, M.A., Price, Q.C. and Leithead, J. (1968). *'Hostels' in Hospital: the analysis of beds in hospital by patient dependency.* Oxford, Oxford University Press for the Nuffield Provincial Hospitals Trust.
10. Townsend, P. (1973). The needs of the elderly and the planning of hospitals. In: *The Needs of the Elderly.* Edited by R.N. Canvin and N.G. Pearson. Exeter, Institute of Biometry and Community Medicine, University of Exeter.
11. Ferguson Anderson (1976). Personal communication.
12. Kay, D.W.K., Beamish, D. and Roth, M. (1964). Old age mental disorder in Newcastle on Tyne. *British Journal of Psychiatry,* **110,** 146.

8

Alternatives to Geriatric Care

J.C. Brocklehurst

In discussing medical practice it is now a cliché to say that the very old form one of the greatest challenges for the rest of the twentieth century. Nevertheless it is true. A growth of 42 per cent in the over 85s in the 20 years 1971-1991 compared with 16 per cent of the over 65s and 8 per cent of the total population; the fact that two-thirds of the disabled are over 75 (1); and that every woman aged 85 and over in Glasgow spends, on average, the last 6 months of her life in hospital (2) – these facts speak for themselves.

Specialist geriatric care has developed progressively in the UK, despite opposition from many quarters and despite generally very poor resources, to such an extent that now there is a structure of geriatric care throughout the land which is second to none in the world.

Present Geriatric Structure

The geriatric service is based on the hospital beds of the consultant (usually 120-150 per consultant, occasionally many more) and these, together with the day hospital, provide a form of progressive patient care with three main elements: acute treatment, rehabilitation and long-term care. About 1 in 10 of patients admitted to the acute geriatric ward ends up as a long-term patient. In most areas the consultant or one of his staff will go and see patients at home before admitting them, to obtain a history, to discuss with relatives the pattern of care required and to suggest alternatives to admission. The geriatrician is a manager of quite considerable resources (though often insufficient for the load he has to carry). He is the leader of a rehabilitation team of nurses, therapists and social workers and, because of the nature of disease in old age, he often has a continuing relationship with his patients, which he shares with the general practitioner, over many years.

Is this system the best? What are the alternatives?

Two often canvassed alternatives are: first, that geriatric medicine should return to the fold of general medicine and disappear as a specialty; second, that general practitioners with their attached social workers and access to community hospitals can provide most of the geriatric service themselves.

Back to General Medicine?

Geriatric medicine began because general physicians neglected the elderly and had little interest in the continuing management of long-term disability in old age. They looked after chronic sick wards, containing many ill-diagnosed and inadequately treated old people who, with greater interest and more care, could have been returned to the community. With few exceptions, there is no evidence to suggest that internists as a body would be any more interested now in the continuing management of disability in old age than they were in the 1940s and before. It is their nature to lose interest when the acute phase of the illness has passed. No doubt a new generation of internists could be trained to accept the challenge of geriatrics but they would do this at the expense of other specialties (cardiac, endocrinological, thoracic, rheumatic, etc.) and would end up as now – geriatricians. Alternatively, perhaps internists could simply deal with the acute phase and pass their patients on to physical medicine specialists for rehabilitation and to someone else if long-term care is required. This is possible if enough doctors would accept specialization in physical medicine and in long-term care but there is no evidence that either of these would be more popular than geriatrics on the scale that is needed (at present there are 300 consultant geriatricians in the UK). As for efficiency and economics, surely one man responsible for the whole process of geriatric care in an individual area will achieve better results than the fragmenting of this among three or more clinicians. Perhaps the greatest shortcoming of medical care of the old in the USA at present is the passing of responsibility from one clinician to another without anyone being concerned for the whole patient throughout the whole period of his disability and rehabilitation. Furthermore, patients would almost certainly prefer to relate to one specialist through this often prolonged and difficult period. It is also certain that one person with an overview of the whole problem will deploy the resources more economically.

General Practitioner as Geriatrician?

The general practitioner alternative founders in the first place on the divided responsibility this would entail for a very expensive commodity in short supply – the long-term hospital bed. Individual general practitioners know the demand from their own practices but cannot possibly assess priorities for care between their own patients and those of the 29 or so other general practitioners who would be using the same facilities. If beds were available for all, the problem would not arise (or might not), but this happy state would be almost profligate when the 'medical pound' is so scarce and has to be spent in so many different ways. Additionally, the practicality of 20 or 30 general practitioners supervising the complex processes of assessment and rehabilitation all within three or four wards and one day hospital would be an administrative – and nursing – nightmare. The expert with overall knowledge of the conflicting needs of disabled old people in one area, born of his responsibility for them, has proved the best system so far and, I believe, appears the most rational.

Practical Alternatives

More attractive alternatives must be sought to individual parts rather than to the whole system. All acute medical and acute geriatric beds should be shared – located together – with the young and old, admitted here under the care of the appropriate physician, cardiologist, endocrinologist, rheumatologist or geriatrician. This would promote better communication and understanding of each other's problems, for the good of all – patient and doctor alike.

Patients, whether young or old, should never be admitted to these wards simply 'for observation and investigation'. In the elderly much observation and investigation can be done in the day hospital or the out-patient clinic. If admission is required for this purpose, it should be well preprogrammed, so that it requires only two or three nights in hospital, possibly with a return in a week or two's time for some additional procedure. The '48-hour bed' is a good concept.

Quite often a deteriorating or highly unstable household (perhaps an 84-year-old stroke patient living with her 65-year-old widowed daughter) can be contained by social support at home, day hospital attendance and periodic short-term admission (for 'relief of relative's strain'). This is well founded geriatric practice. But the short-term admission bed should be prebooked – so that it is continuously programmed and so that individual situations are boosted at regular enough intervals to forestall collapse.

How much geriatric medicine can be undertaken by less highly trained personnel than doctors? Some argue that preadmission assessment visits could be carried out by social workers or nurses. If the purpose of such a visit were simply to assess the social problem (and there nearly always is one) or to discover whether nursing support would contain the situation (a decision the general practitioner will already have made), then this alternative might be arguable. But the preadmission assessment has much more important implications. It is the key encounter between the patient and his relatives and the geriatrician. Decisions made at this time on medical as well as social evidence will influence the whole subsequent programme of the patient's management. Neither nurse nor social worker (as at present trained) is fitted for this role.

One role which very clearly suggests itself for a particular nurse – the health visitor – is the ascertainment of unreported illness. Old people at present don't report a lot of their problems to general practitioners. They ascribe them to their age and believe that nothing can be done. Williamson and his colleagues (3), and many others since then, have shown much remediable morbidity in old age (for example, impaired vision, hearing and walking; unrecognized anaemia; depression; dementia; and urinary problems) which is unreported and therefore untreated. The health-centre-based health visitor with the practice age/sex register at hand is the ideal person to discover this unreported morbidity and arrange for its treatment. A practice list of 3,000 will contain, on average, 270 patients aged over 70. If the health visitor devotes one afternoon a week to this task she could see, examine and counsel all the patients over 70 on the practice list in 12-18 months. This does make good economic sense.

Residential (Part 3) homes have a clientele which overlaps that of the geriatric long-term care wards. Why not therefore develop more long-term care within local authority homes (which are cheaper) rather than hospitals (which are more expensive)? Certainly, the local authority homes have successfully developed a suitable environment for the care of frail old people who must be looked after for the rest of their lives, and this the hospital service has signally failed to do. The universal fact of having to spend the last years of your life sleeping and living in a communal space with anything from 5 to 39 other individuals is a distasteful way of life which is not imposed even in penal institutions. Only long-term hospitals (and some public schools) retain this archaic enforced communality. Residential homes long ago replaced open dormitories with single or, at the most, double bedrooms. In this regard they would certainly be much better places for long-term geriatric patients to live in than the present hospitals.

However, there are two considerable problems in transferring geriatric care to residential homes. First, the homes would have to increase the numbers and change the training of their staffs, with emphasis on nursing. While geriatric and Part 3 residents are all part of a continuum, the geriatric patients are, as a class, the most disabled and mentally impaired. In making these staff changes, the cost of the residential home would become the same as that of the hospital. However, if the environment were so much better, what matter? The other problem is that as mini-hospitals they might be too small, but this is a conjecture. When is a hospital too small? Empirical evidence would suggest when the bed provision falls below 60 or 70, but this is opinion.

It is clear that Part 3 and geriatric long-term residents have in common a degree of frailty and dependency, and for this reason the whole of this area of supportive care might better be the responsibility of the geriatric service. All should have the single bedrooms with lounge, dining room, studio and garden found in most good residential homes. It may be argued whether this complex should or should not be on the hospital campus (district general or community hospital). However, this is a matter which is unlikely to affect the economics of the actual care which is given.

The emphasis of social (as distinct from medical) care should be within the increasing development of sheltered housing – where our money is being properly spent at the present time. Sheltered housing groups might profitably be linked with day centres, allowing a restaurant to be used by the sheltered housing residents as well as by those old people living in their own homes in the neighbourhood.

Euthanasia

One aspect of old age where an alternative approach is often urged, is in relation to medical treatment at the end of life and the concept of euthanasia. It is sometimes suggested that there are possible alternatives to geriatric care which are moral and are economically attractive. The geriatric and psychogeriatric services have three main functions. The first is to consider all the factors relevant to breakdown in an old person's living – involving accurate diagnosis, preceded by careful investigation and followed by rational therapy; the second is rehabilitation to promote maximum possible independence and to maintain the patient living in the community for as long as is possible; the third is the humane and sympathetic care of those old people who are so disabled as to need to spend the last months or years of their lives in long-term care. This third group includes many sensible physically disabled old people, together with many at all stages of dementia, with or without physical disability. It is in this last group that suggestions are made that doctors should cut life short (and similar arguments have been made in relation to patients in mental subnormality hospitals). If such lives are not to be shortened, it is suggested that at least they should not be prolonged artificially.

I am certain that no doctor practising in the UK would ever consider it his responsibility to cut short a patient's life. It is unthinkable. It would amount to homicide, which is a criminal offence. If a patient in sound mind requests it, it would be euthanasia (or homicide on request) and it is this aspect of a doctor's involvement which has some vociferous proponents, although few of them within the profession itself. The demand for euthanasia comes from those who apply it to themselves in the future, not in the present. Few of those who are old and in sound mind ever ask a doctor to end their lives; and when they do it is usually for one of three reasons: they are suffering from depression (which needs treatment); they are overwhelmed by distressing symptoms (pain, nausea, breathlessness) which it is the doctor's responsibility to relieve and which it is almost always in his power to relieve; or they feel a burden to their relatives. In this last case, if the burden is real and not a fantasy it can usually be relieved by sharing it. But no doctor is likely to accept the role of executioner, and the health and well-being of the profession of medicine depends on such a refusal. That doctors should involve themselves in senicide or dementicide is also unthinkable.

However, what about keeping people alive by artificial means – a different but no less complex problem? It is a problem of two dimensions. First there is the human dimension; that is, what is the quality of life – can we assess it for another person, and, if so, can we allow ourselves to put a lower limit to that which is acceptable? The second is the economic dimension – that of some patients being denied life-maintaining resources which they need, because these resources are being unreasonably deployed with others. Certainly some old people at present die while awaiting hospital admission and if this waiting time is significant then the only alternatives are either to devote more resources to the management of the old or to withdraw some from those whose quality of life seems to be irreversibly deteriorated below a lower limit. The only resource which is really in question here (that is in relation to the old) is the staffed hospital bed. Respirators, artificial kidneys and the other complex and scarce life-maintaining resources are hardly ever used with the very old – and this is arguably correct. On the other hand, antibiotics and other more readily available therapeutic procedures may prolong life and thus continue the occupancy of staffed hospital beds. Whether or not to use antibiotics in infection in demented old people is a personal decision in which the physician has little guidance other than his own humanity and experience to fall back on. Often, of course, it is the youngest and least experienced doctor who has to make the decision – in the evening or at night.

One thing that must not be lost sight of is that patients have every right to refuse treatment, and this right must be upheld.

Miscellaneous Propositions

Finally, this consideration of alternatives to geriatric care may state, rather than assess, a number of miscellaneous propositions.

Are Junior Medical Staff Really Necessary? Clearly there are many more junior appointments in the British hospital service than are needed for training purposes. Is there any justification for retaining them and so perpetuating a hospital career structure which is pyramidal, wasteful and often a despair to those in the lower and broader part of the pyramid? In the USA many hospitals are run successfully without junior doctors. The consultants (or specialists) would then be more involved with the patient at every stage. Fewer investigations would be carried out and decisions would be more rapidly and effectively translated into action. I think it is likely that a team of three to five consultant geriatricians with good nursing and technical support might well function much more effectively without the interposition of junior medical staff. In such a situation, training posts (including preregistration internships) would be provided only for training purposes.

Multidisciplinary Madness? Geriatric practice is firmly based on team work involving physicians, nurses, therapists and social workers, each making an essential contribution. Currently, however, there seems to be a danger of this principle being carried to extremes, all having to be represented at every stage of planning and decision-making and all spending much too much time involved in the work of others. This is probably linked with the current tendency in the National Health Service for clinicians to become committee men. Doctors are trained to treat patients and are most effectively employed when they do this. Nowadays committees often come before clinics. Perhaps the only way to overcome this and to ensure that only the vitally interested and thus those who have a real contribution to make are involved in planning committees, is to hold such committees out of the normal hours of work; that is, from 8.00 to 9.00 am, at lunch time or after 5.00 pm.

The Disappearing Chemist. Apparently one chemist shop is closing each day in Great Britain at the present time. Outside urban areas this makes it increasingly difficult for the old to have their prescriptions dispensed and this fact, added to the problems of isolated old people without telephones coping with general practitioners' appointment systems and transporting themselves to health centres, must deter many from obtaining the treatment they need. Some radical rethinking of the supply of medicines to old people (and the disabled) is required.

Inflexible Specialism. Another real human and economic problem affecting the old is the inability of the Health Service to respond quickly to new and advanced therapies for chronic disability. A good example arises in relation to hip replacement operations which can relieve much dependency among a number of the elderly but which are so limited in certain parts of the country by a shortage of orthopaedic surgeons and operating theatres as to produce waiting lists of 18 months or more. These almost automatically rule out the old from serious consideration. A Health Service which was more sensitive to the changing needs of patients would train the specialists who are really needed in their own time and provide them with appropriate resources. This would make economic good sense. We are probably still training too many young doctors in the medically 'popular' specialties, whose skills are not going to be needed (to the great future frustration of these young doctors as they attempt to climb the ladder in that specialty).

Geriatric medicine still ranks as one of the 'less popular' specialties. This is not because of its irrelevance – for it becomes more relevant each year that passes – nor because of its intrinsic lack of clinical interest, for the medicine of the whole man in old age is rich in intellectual and human rewards; but rather because of the perpetuation, through the attitudes of a fortunately diminishing number of senior doctors, of discouragement towards this branch of medicine. Medical students and young doctors can now see the challenge and relevance of medicine in old age – and the future of geriatric medicine, while subsuming many alterations in detail, is firmly founded in its general philosophy for the future.

References

1. Harris, A. (1971). *Handicapped and Impaired in Great Britain*. London, HMSO.
2. Isaacs, B., Livingstone, M. and Neville, Y. (1972). *Survival of the Unfittest*. London and Boston, Routledge and Kegan Paul.
3. Williamson, J., Stokoe, I.H., Gray, S., Fisher, M., Smith, A., McGhee, A. and Stephenson, E. (1964). Old people at home – their unreported needs. *Lancet*, i, 1117-1120.

9

The Painful Facts

R.E. Kendell

Forty years ago when Beveridge was drawing up his plans for a National Health Service, sickness, or ill health, was regarded as a fairly straightforward phenomenon, a temporary and easily recognizable departure from a natural state of health. People 'caught' infections or 'succumbed' to diseases. Sometimes they died but usually they recovered within a few weeks, or at most a few months. Only occasionally did they remain ill for months or years on end. Proper treatment, particularly with the wonderful new drugs such as penicillin and the sulphonamides that were then being discovered, greatly increased and strengthened the natural defences of the body. It seemed reasonable to assume, therefore, that in the future illnesses would, on the whole, be shorter and less severe; fewer people would die and fewer would become chronic invalids. It was taken for granted that only a small minority of the population was ill at any time, and assumed that the total quantity of illness would be reduced steadily as effective treatment became more widely available and the healing powers of modern medicine increased.

These were the assumptions on which the NHS was launched on July 5th 1948. It was recognized, to be sure, that in the first few years demand on the service would be heavy. There would be a great backlog of illness that had formerly gone untreated because people had been unable to afford doctors' fees, and some of these illnesses would have become chronic because treatment had not been instituted early enough. But once this backlog had been dealt with the need for medical services would fall as the population became healthier and illnesses were treated at an earlier stage and with more effective drugs. As a result, so it was thought, the cost to the Exchequer would eventually fall and in time fewer doctors would probably be needed. Indeed, in 1957 the Willink Committee advised a reduction in the intake to medical schools.

When the cost rose year by year instead of falling, and the queues of patients in general practitioners' surgeries and out-patient departments showed no sign of diminishing, both the politicians and the medical profession were puzzled. It seemed clear though that all, or nearly all, of these unexpected patients were genuinely ill and there was no doubting the popularity of the service with the electorate. So it was assumed, without any radical rethinking of the initial assumptions about the nature of ill health, that there must have been more undetected illness in the population than anyone had suspected. More money was pumped into the Health Service, the number of doctors and nurses working in hospitals rose steadily to more than double their 1949 levels and the drug bill rose more than fourfold. The total cost of the Health Service rose from £477 million in 1950 to £2,083 million in 1970 and to £3,603 million in 1974.

Part of this massive increase in expenditure and medical manpower was devoted to campaigns to identify undetected or presymptomatic illness – routine chest x-rays to detect undiagnosed tuberculosis or neoplasms, routine cervical smears to detect carcinoma of the cervix, screening programmes for diabetes and hypertension, 'well baby' clinics and the like. Most of it, however, was simply a response to a steadily increasing demand from the general population for more and better facilities across the whole spectrum of medical care. It was only towards the end of the 1960s that people began to comment on some disturbing features of this massive enterprise, and to question the basic assumptions of the original architects. The most obvious problem was the way in which demand always increased to outstrip supply. The more general practitioners a community obtained, the higher the community's consultation rate became; the more surgeons and out-patient clinics a regional board provided in an attempt to reduce its waiting lists, the more patients were transferred to hospital by their GPs. In 1949 there were 497,700 people on waiting lists for admission to hospital; in 1969, despite the enormous increase in expenditure and in hospital admission rates that had taken place in the interim, there were 561,365 (1).

It was also increasingly clear that the new drugs and technologies which were becoming available were not only more powerful but also more expensive than anyone had anticipated. And that, rather than curing people, all too often these treatments merely kept alive as chronic invalids people who would formerly have died: children with spina bifida, adults with renal failure, and the paralysed or demented survivors of car crashes. Even more disconcerting was the fact that there was little evidence that the population was becoming significantly healthier as a result of all this effort and expenditure. The number of working days lost through sickness was 281 million in 1954. By 1970 the number of days lost had actually risen to 342 million. Infant mortality rates had fallen, but they had fallen less than in many other countries and the rate of fall was declining steadily. Life expectancy at birth had risen by no more than a year or two between 1948 and 1968 and for men of 60 or over it had actually declined. No commercial enterprise could ever survive such disastrous performance figures without the most searching examination of its objectives, its management and its market, and it is no coincidence that the people to draw attention to these unwholesome facts were mainly economists and administrators rather than patients, politicians or doctors.

The public, by and large, was satisfied with its Health Service. There were grumbles about hospital waiting lists and hospital food, and recurrent complaints about the lack of specialized facilities for relatively uncommon conditions like chronic renal failure and infantile autism, but most people seemed content with the medical care they received and fondly imagined that their weekly National Insurance contributions were paying the whole cost of the NHS rather than a tiny fraction of it (6.3 per cent in 1974). Politicians were alarmed by the inexorably mounting cost of the service but its central objective – 'to meet health needs wherever and whenever they arise' without financial or other deterrents – was too sacred to the Labour Party for any detached appraisal to be feasible in that quarter, and their Conservative counterparts were too well aware of the electoral dangers involved to do more than introduce a few minor charges to patients and talk of increased managerial efficiency. The medical profession, and the other health care professions with it, simply demanded more money and more and better facilities for itself and its patients. Indeed, the demand for expansion, and the insistence that existing staffing levels and facilities were inadequate, had come from the medical profession rather than the electorate itself all along. Politicians and planners both accepted that the assessment of 'health needs' was a medical responsibility, and for the most part doctors accepted that the patients who came to their surgeries and out-patient clinics were in need of treatment. As they were already working at full stretch it seemed self-evident that this treatment could not be provided unless the service was expanded. As a former Minister of Health once observed, 'one of the most striking features of the NHS is the continual, deafening chorus of complaint which rises day and night from every part of it' (2).

The central problem, which we are only just beginning to grasp, is that neither the 'demand' for medical care (expressed by patients) or the 'need' (perceived by doctors) is finite, or even a function of a finite quantity of sickness in the community. Both are potentially infinite, and regulated not so much by the health or sickness of the population as by the actual level of provision of services. The Health Service has been failing to meet the demands placed upon it because, like the Norse god Thor, its staff have been trying to drink dry a vessel whose tip lies beneath the sea.

The fact is that dis-ease of one kind or another is so widespread as to be almost universal. Wadsworth and his colleagues (3) found that 95 per cent of those they surveyed in Bermondsey and Southwark considered themselves to have been unwell during the preceding 14 days. Dunnell and Cartwright (4) likewise found only 5 per cent of their respondents completely symptom free over a similar period, and 9 per cent claimed to have suffered more than six different symptoms during that period. North American studies have produced similar findings. Clearly, headaches, coughs and colds, aches and pains, and feelings of depression and tension are so widespread that to be without them for long is abnormal. At the present time most people do not usually consult doctors when they develop these symptoms, though many more do so than 20 years ago. They endure them, or treat them themselves with analgesics or proprietary remedies, for a variety of reasons – because they don't want to 'waste the doctor's time' or to waste their own time sitting in his surgery, or because they do not yet regard it as a doctor's job to treat emotional problems or relatively minor bodily symptoms.

But a patient's concept of a doctor's role, and his own concept too, can change considerably from one generation to the next, and is largely determined by his availability. If doctors are scarce and expensive, they are usually only consulted about serious or life-threatening illnesses. If their availability increases, and it costs nothing to visit them, people consult them about less serious conditions, and both the patient's and the doctor's concept of his proper role change accordingly. We have seen this happening quite rapidly in the last 30 years, and if availability continues to increase both lay and medical concepts of a doctor's role will continue to change. If there were more general practitioners, for example, they would have more time to listen to their patients' complaints and would be able to do more for the unhappy, the bereaved, the lonely and the frustrated, to say nothing of young men with minor sporting injuries, gardeners with backache and girls with dysmenorrhoea. In other words, increased availability would lead inexorably to new demands from patients, a further expansion of both lay and medical concepts of the doctor's role, and hence to further demands for more doctors.

Despite the protests of Ivan Illich and some other lone voices at what they see as the medicalization of social problems and an enfeebling dependence on a vast 'healthocracy' governing our lives from conception to the grave, to most people, and to many doctors, this is not an unpleasing or an alarming prospect (5, 6). It is doubtful, though, whether it is a viable one. The National Health Service already employs nearly a million people, over 5 per cent of the total work-force. If one considers the competing claims of education, transport and other public services, and the urgent need to decrease the proportion of the work-force engaged on wealth-consuming rather than wealth-producing activities, it is doubtful whether this figure can or should be increased any further. The nation already sends each year over 3,500 of its most able university entrants to medical schools to train as doctors, and the number will rise to 3,945 by 1980. As the academic standards required for admission to medical schools are higher than those required by any other university faculty, it may be pertinent to ask whether we may already be allowing too high a proportion of our most talented school leavers to go into medicine.

These facts have to be stated and these questions asked not merely because of the nation's current economic difficulties, or because of the urgent need to reduce public spending for the next few years. Essentially the same problems face, or will soon face, much wealthier countries also. Regardless of whether health services are financed by private insurance or by central government revenues, and almost regardless of the gross national product, the point must come, long before either demand or need have been satisfied, at which any further expansion of health services in terms of money or manpower can only take place at the expense of other equally important public services, or at the risk of weakening the economy as a whole. It is, of course, true that several countries already spend a higher proportion of their gross national product on their health services than we do in the UK. Dollar for dollar the USA spends three times as much. But it is not obvious that they are any healthier as a result. Indeed it could be argued quite plausibly that, over all, the NHS provides its citizens with as high a standard of health care as any other country and at considerably lower cost – the financial saving being effected mainly by underpaying nurses, doctors and paraclinical staff of all kinds. If the nation's economic fortunes were to improve dramatically over the next decade, it is doubtful whether the service provided to the community would improve very much, and even more doubtful whether any objective index of the nation's health would show any improvement. Wages and salaries account for 69 per cent of the total NHS budget and the greater part of any increase in that budget in an era of rising prosperity would inevitably be swallowed by wage and salary rises for existing employees, leaving comparatively little for new buildings, new staff or new equipment.

These two facts – the fact that the demand for medical services, and the need as doctors perceive it, will always exceed the supply, and the fact that supply in terms of cost and manpower must already be at or close to the limits of what is feasible – carry with them profound implications for medicine. They mean that everything the NHS provides is provided at the expense of something else for which there is also a demand, or a potential demand, and which is necessary, or at least desirable, on medical grounds. At a more personal level, they mean that every patient one treats is treated at the expense of some other perhaps equally deserving patient; that every time one devotes additional time or resources to one patient, another potential patient is deprived of that time or those resources; and that every time one succeeds in obtaining new accommodation or more staff for one's own clinical team or one's own specialty, the community is deprived of something else, perhaps a geriatric day centre, or a renal dialysis unit, or more nurses and psychologists in a mental deficiency hospital. Until recently we have all evaded, or failed to see, this uncomfortable dilemma. This was partly because we didn't realize that, in clamouring for the staff and resources necessary to provide what we regarded as adequate treatment for the ever increasing numbers of patients attending our surgeries and out-patient clinics, we were seeking the impossible. It was also because we were slow to appreciate that the ethical obligations of a physician working in a health service are different from those of private practice.

In the past – 30 years ago, 100 years ago, even 2,000 years ago – a doctor's duty had always been to his patient: the invalid in his consulting room, the sick child whose parents had summoned him, the men and women lying in his ward. There were occasions, to be sure, when physicians were swamped with conflicting demands they could not begin to meet; in time of war, during epidemics, in the aftermath of disasters of all kinds. But for most of the time, even though disease and sickness might be rife in the population at large, it was accepted that the physician's obligation was to the patients whom he was treating or who were actively seeking his services. For them, provided they could recompense him adequately for his time and his skill, no effort was too great, no course of treatment too long or too expensive. He was at their service, and had no obligations to anyone else.

But in a situation in which everyone, by virtue of the taxes he has paid or others have paid on his behalf, has the same right to medical care, and individual doctors are responsible for providing a service to a population, rather than merely to the individuals who gain access to them, the priorities and the ethical issues are changed. Just as the general practitioner has an obligation to all those who are registered with him, whether they come to his surgery or not, so the physician or surgeon has an obligation to all the inhabitants of the catchment area of his hospital; not just to those in his ward or his out-patient clinic. Both, therefore, have to adopt whatever course seems most likely to be of greatest benefit to the health of the population they are responsible for; and they have to do so with their existing resources. The days when we could aspire to give everyone the treatment we felt he needed without regard to the financial implications, and to demand more staff and more equipment to enable us to do so, are over. We have learnt that we will never be able to do all the things we want to, and that we will always be forced to choose. Either we can treat one patient in the way we would like to, and leave another untreated, or we can treat both in a way we regard as second best. But we cannot treat both in the way we would like to. And if the time ever does come when we have enough resources to do so, assuredly by then there will be three patients waiting to be treated, or else our conception of what constitutes adequate treatment will have become more comprehensive and more expensive in the interim.

To me this is the real ethical dilemma of modern medicine, because it colours the clinical decisions one makes every day. The moral dilemmas posed by euthanasia, abortion, artificial insemination and the prolongation of irreversible coma by mechanical ventilators are real enough, but most of the time most doctors do not need to worry about them. The knowledge that whenever one treats one patient, one is thereby either directly or indirectly depriving someone else affects, or should affect, nearly every clinical decision one makes.

If it is always a choice between doing A and doing B, and if clamouring for the resources to do both is unrealistic and ultimately dishonest, it is clear that we must do everything in our power to make the right choices. We must know how effective each of the treatments at our disposal really is, and what the total cost, direct and indirect, of each of them is as well. We are all used to comparing the efficacy of different treatments. Economists are also well used to comparing the costs of alternative strategies. But only recently have attempts been made to combine the two and analyse both the cost and the benefits simultaneously. It has been shown, for example, that the treatment of varicose veins by injection and compression as an out-patient is usually just as effective as stripping under general anaesthesia as an in-patient, and considerably cheaper to both the Health Service and the patient (7). It has also been shown fairly convincingly that renal transplantation is both a cheaper and a more effective treatment for chronic renal failure than dialysis (8). Even straightforward comparisons such as these inevitably involve many approximations and arbitrary assumptions. It was assumed in the renal failure comparison, for example, that the quality of life while undergoing regular dialysis was only 0.75 of that after successful transplantation, and it is remarkably difficult to calculate the total cost, direct and indirect, to either the patient or the Health Service of even quite simple procedures. It will obviously be far harder to compare the costs and benefits of treating different conditions – screening for cancer of the cervix by cervical cytology compared with screening for cancer of the breast by mammography, for example. But, however difficult such comparisons may be and however many arbitrary assumptions have to be made in the process, choice is unavoidable. As economists have emphasized, the only open issue is whether these choices are made wittingly or unwittingly, and to believe that cost-benefit analysis is unnecessary or impossible is to assume that unwitting decisions are likely to be better than witting ones (9).

However, even if, by a rigorous application of cost-benefit analysis, we restrict ourselves to the cheapest and most effective treatments, and even if increasing national prosperity enables us to spend more money and devote even more personnel to health services than we do already, neither the demand nor the need will ever be satisfied. In the long run the problem can only be solved by a change in public and medical attitudes to health and disease. In the end, we and our patients both have to accept, as mankind always accepted in the past, not only that death is inevitable but also that some degree of dis-ease during life is also inevitable. We have to accept that medicine can never eliminate depression, ennui and frustration. We have to accept that the World Health Organization's definition of health as 'a state of complete physical, mental and social well being' is pie in the sky and always will be.

It is comparatively easy for economists, administrators and epidemiologists to accept the logic of this argument and to lecture clinicians on the need for realism and financial discipline. It is far, far harder for clinicians to do so faced with queues of deserving patients in their out-patient clinics and knowing how much more they could achieve if they had sufficient time and resources. And it must be harder still for the patient himself. But in the long run we will all have to face the facts, for ignoring them will not cause them to fade away. It is easier to rail against untrustworthy politicians and incompetent administrators than to change deeply rooted attitudes and aspirations, but sooner or later change we must. If we thought more deeply about our priorities we could achieve much more than we do. An important part of the problem, of course, is that the branches of medicine which command the highest prestige, and the therapeutic activities which attract the most talented members of each new generation of doctors and establish their reputations for them, are generally those whose cost effectiveness is lowest. Open heart surgery, coronary care units packed with electronic gadgetry and long-term psychotherapy, for example. It will not be easy for us to forego the challenges and excitements of these activities and concentrate our energies on the immunization of babies, the fluoridation of water supplies and the development of an effective out-patient treatment for haemorrhoids. But sooner or later we must.

References

1. Cooper, M.H. (1975). *Rationing Health Care.* London, Croom Helm.
2. Powell, E. (1966). *Medicine and Politics.* London, Pitman.
3. Wadsworth, M.E.J., Blaney, R. and Butterfield, W.J.H. (1971). *Health and Sickness: the Choice of Treatment.* London, Tavistock.
4. Dunnell, K. and Cartwright, A. (1972). *Medicine Takers, Prescribers and Hoarders.* London, Routledge & Kegan Paul.
5. Illich, I. (1975). *Medical Nemesis.* London, Calder & Boyars.
6. Office of Health Economics (1975). *The Health Care Dilemma,* London, OHE.
7. Piachaud, D. and Weddell, J.M. (1972). *International Journal of Epidemiology,* **1**, 287.
8. Klarman, H.E., Francis, J.O'S. and Rosenthal, G.D. (1968). *Medical Care,* **6**, 48.
9. Williams, A. (1974). *British Medical Bulletin,* **30**, 252.

Part Two
Diagnosis and Decision Making

10

The Science of Diagnosis

E.J. Moran Campbell

In this chapter I shall be concerned with diagnosis, the noun – the terms we apply to illnesses – and the verb – the process of deciding which terms to apply. I shall discuss them from a scientific viewpoint which is popularly called 'Popperian' (1, 2).

Diagnosis, the Noun

In particular what do we mean by 'a disease'? I think doctors should use diagnostic terms in the same way as scientists use technical terms. This way is well put by Popper when he points out that most scientific statements should be read from right to left rather than from left to right.

'A di-neutron is an unstable system comprising two neutrons', is a scientist's answer to the question, 'what shall we call an unstable system comprising two neutrons?', not an answer to the question, 'what is a di-neutron?'. The word di-neutron is a handy substitute for a long description, that is all; no information about physics is to be gained from analysing it.' (3)

To use philosophical jargon, the scientist is a nominalist, not an essentialist.

I believe the same use of words should be true of medicine. The labels we use in medicine should be read from right to left and not from left to right. Much difficulty in communication, both in practice and in research, stems from an implicit belief that an 'essence' lies behind our labels. Let me risk the example of asthma. Five years ago a group of experts were unable to agree on an 'identification' or 'definition' of asthma (4). I was not there but, having read the proceedings and spoken to many of the participants, I believe the failure was due to the fact that enough of those present could not accept a definition which did not accord with their preconception of the 'essentials' of the disease called asthma. To them the issue was more fundamental than the reshaping of a verbal tool which, due to changing circumstances and advances in understanding, is no longer doing its job very well.

What do we Mean by 'a Disease'? I think the best definition so far put forward is as follows: 'The sum of the abnormal phenomena displayed by a group of living organisms in association with a specified common characteristic or characteristics by which they differ from the norm for their species in such a way as to place them at a biological disadvantage' (5).

This is clearly a nominalist definition but does it coincide with usage? It seems to me that much of our teaching implies that patients become ill because they are attacked by a disease and in deciding which disease we face a fairly straightforward case in determining class membership in accordance with the rules of logic. The ideal abstract classes are mutually exclusive and jointly exhaustive. In the eighteenth century when the concept of diseases seems to have been unequivocally essentialist, both De Sauvages and (perhaps not surprisingly!) Linnaeus produced classifications of the diseases 'then known' (6). In the nineteenth century the discovery of micro-organisms and the authoritative descriptions of diseases on a basis of morbid anatomy reinforced this essentialist view. But since then our understanding has proceeded in many different directions so that our classifications today are really heterologous lists.

Let me take a different tack and suggest that another way of looking at a disease is as a paradigm in one of the senses that Kuhn (7) uses the term. At its simplest, as reflected in our teaching and in the composition of most textbooks, the paradigm of a disease is as follows.

A disease is first recognized syndromally – a constellation of clinical features. The disease has a cause (infective, nutritional, genetic, immunological, etc.); this cause produces characteristic structural changes, which in turn produce the clinical manifestations. The elucidation of the causative, structural and functional changes may not come in any particular historical order but the paradigm has two characteristics: first, it is expected or at least hoped that the relations will be specific (unique cause, unique structural and functional changes belonging to one syndrome); second, as knowledge progresses, the defining characteristic is 'pushed to the left' in the sequence given above. In other words, a disease will not be left in syndromal terms if it can be explained or defined in functional terms; a functional syndrome will not be left in these terms if it can be characterized structurally and 'cause' takes priority over all. As witness, I would cite the avoidance of the term 'disease' when, from the beginning, such specificity is unlikely (e.g. malabsorption syndrome, respiratory distress syndrome) or if it turns out not to be true (e.g. the demotion of angina pectoris from a disease to a syndrome).

I am now going to develop a whimsical metaphor that the oncogeny of the diagnosis of the individual patient recapitulates the phylogeny of medical scientific history, using the example of asthma. Two thousand years ago a Greek who went to his physician complaining of being wakened at night by breathlessness would be told that he had been afflicted by asthma. He might further be told that young people suffering from this affliction tend to grow out of it but that in older people it is often followed by the dropsy and early death.

Let us now leap ahead to the beginning of this century and play the scene again assuming that our physician thinks pathophysiologically rather as we do today. The physician elicits evidence that the patient either has evidence of air-flow obstruction or of indistensible congested lungs. He will therefore (in 1900) diagnose either bronchial asthma or cardiac asthma. Let us pursue the second of these first. The physician believes that there is a back pressure from the heart causing congestion of the lungs and so on. Let us assume he finds high blood pressure and then the story is complete; the end-point is reached – the diagnosis (disease) is hypertension. (Although, of course, the famous Pickering - Platt controversy could be cited as evidence that the question whether or not hypertension is a disease remains open.) Since 1900 progress has been such that cardiac asthma is no longer an end-point, a diagnosis, a disease. Indeed, it is no longer even a useful staging point en route to diagnosis or a useful term in scientific discourse. So, in about 1950, it begins to disappear from the books.

But what about bronchial asthma? We have been accumulating lots of information (clinical, environmental, allergic, immunological, pharmacological, physiological, histological, etc.), but instead of letting the word asthma adapt in some agreed way to the shifting situation we either expect the cause of the disease to be revealed or argue about its nature.

An Experimental Study of the Usage of the Term 'Disease'. I tried to design an experiment to test the hypothesis that acceptance of a diagnostic term as meaning a disease conformed with the hierarchy (mentioned above) in which cause takes priority over structure, which in turn takes priority over function, which in turn takes priority over syndrome. I hoped to get a quantitative assessment of the need doctors feel to have information about cause in their diagnostic terms before calling them diseases. I hoped that the need would not be great but I was doubtful.

I will not go through my early studies in detail. In brief, I compiled a list of 60 terms which might be accepted as diseases in a matrix with several body systems or subspecialties on one axis and the 'field of study' (cause, structure, function, syndrome) from which it seemed likely that the most useful defining characteristic for each of them might be selected on the other. Table 10.1 gives a selection of the results. In the first column are those terms which 95 per cent of the doctors I studied called diseases. So the idea was supported that real diseases are those in which a satisfactory

Table 10.1
Is it a disease?

More than 95% 'Yes'	*50 - 70% 'Yes'*	*Less than 50% 'Yes'*
Measles	Hypertension	Traumatic paraplegia
Syphilis	Epilepsy	Chronic mountain sickness
Whooping cough	Cirrhosis	Multiple traumatic fractures
Amoebic dysentery	Tabes	Accidental hypothermia
Tuberculosis	Asthma	Motor vehicle accident
Gluten-induced enteropathy		

statement of cause is stated or is implied. Indeed tuberculosis and syphilis are statements about little else unless one specifies what organ or system is affected. It was also encouraging to note the readiness to accept such terms as hypertension and epilepsy as diseases.

However, I had also included the terms shown in the third column. These all scored less than 50 per cent. Like the high scorers, these terms can be defining causally within the framework of Scadding's general description of 'a disease'. It seems that one difference between the high and low scorers is in the nature of the cause: injuries, events or physical agents are not regarded as diseases and reference to them in a diagnostic term precludes the condition to which they refer from being regarded as a disease.

Table 10.2
Is it a disease — stage 2

More than half of both groups said 'Yes'	*Doctors*	*School-boys*	*More than half the doctors said 'Yes' Less than half the schoolboys said 'Yes'*	*Doctors*	*School-boys*
Measles	100	95	Lead poisoning	84	28
Poliomyelitis	99	94	CO poisoning	67	15
Malaria	99	95	Gallstones	67	49
Syphilis	99	98	Piles	67	49
Haemophilia	98	93	Heatstroke	63	12
Tuberculosis	98	98	Alcoholism	62	48
Schizophrenia	96	52	Barbiturate overdose	59	10
Cancer of the lung	95	98	Fractured skull	59	3
Diabetes	95	89	Tennis elbow	56	20
Multiple sclerosis	90	95	Depression	56	19
			Hypertension	54	34
Duodenal ulcer	84	53			
Pneumonia	84	79	*Less than half of either group said 'Yes'*		
Emphysema	82	84			
Coronary thrombosis	82	77	Malnutrition	31	29
Acne	77	65	Colour blindness	38	37
			Drowning	31	3
Cirrhosis	77	91	High blood pressure	45	32
Asthma	73	75			
Hay fever	73	62	Hangover	22	2
Muscular dystrophy	73	88	Starvation	18	12
Epilepsy	53	68	Senility	14	29

This tentative conclusion led me to think that the issue has a cultural aspect which is as important as the intellectual or semantic aspect. This cultural aspect may depend on the 'primitive' need to have agencies or explanations for illnesses when no event or overt external agency was apparent to the patient. To test this idea I developed a list of terms that are known to non-medical as well as medical people. So far, I have done the experiment on a group of sixth form schoolboys (n = 106) and a group of academic medical doctors (n = 126). Table 10.2 is a selection from the results.

The interim conclusion seems to be supported. If we assume that the schoolboys become the doctors then it seems that they move towards a more nominalist position but their cultural background holds them back and on occasion is dominant. One cannot help speculating about the reason doctors were so much readier to accept certain terms as diseases (e.g. lead poisoning and fracture of the skull) than others (e.g. hangover and starvation). It seems they are more likely to call a condition a disease if they see some role for themselves in its management.

So What? Does this ambivalent use of diagnostic terms matter? I think it does, both in practice and in research.

First, in practice, it can be unfortunate if a patient who has had a label applied to him by one doctor who uses it just as a label, is then treated by another doctor to whom it means something different – a demon or causative agent to be eradicated by some specific treatment. Secondly, in research, it is confusing if people try to separate the inseparable. Let me risk an example: the field of the connective tissue disorders. At present I do not think we have any right to assume that these diseases, as currently diagnosed, are strictly separable in any fundamental causative sense; nor that the distinction between them lies in the same field of study. Thus it seems to me that rheumatoid arthritis is still a syndrome. Systemic lupus erythematosus seems to some people to be best defined syndromally, to some histologically and, to an increasing number, immunologically. Polyarteritis nodosa and giant cell arteritis seem to be defined structurally; but even here the criteria seem to be different in that polyarteritis nodosa is characterized by the distribution of the lesions whereas giant cell arteritis is characterized by cell type.

I am not denying that typical cases show clusters of features but I doubt that we can say they represent the results of quite distinct agencies or that the typical case can define the marginal. I am not disputing the practical implications of trying to decide whether a particular patient 'has rheumatoid arthritis or SLE' because the hidden purpose of such discussions is of course the probability that the patient will have a good or a bad prognosis, will or will not develop renal trouble, will or will not be likely to need steroids. But I believe we should avoid being misled into accepting the implication that there are separate demons called rheumatoid arthritis and SLE. Indeed, one may be better off looking at the clusters of features for guidance, without forcing patients into disease entities. Information may well be lost. When present at such clinical discussions I sometimes feel like an agnostic at an ecumenical meeting: I share the wish to do good but doubt the need for the doctrinal discussions.

Unless we are able to distinguish between diseases in terms of features derived from the same field of study, we may be wasting our time asking 'either - or' type questions and our classifications are liable to be mixed up lists. I think it is incumbent upon us to adopt a nominalist position while recognizing that for much of ordinary clinical discourse we will have to accept the hidden implications of old habits. However, the physicist or engineer seems to be able to use words like force, work or energy technically without confusion with colloquial usage.

Diagnosis, the Verb – the Diagnostic Process

For several years I have been concerned that we make the acquisition of diagnostic ability unnecessarily difficult because we teach what we were brainwashed into thinking we should do rather than what we actually do. Like others (8) I have been struck by the applicability of Popper's views of the nature of scientific enquiry to the diagnostic process, and I would like to put this belief in some explicit form which might be of practical use in teaching.

My concern, however, has another reason beyond making it easier to become a doctor. I believe that everybody – patients, doctors and tax-payers – should have an interest in a more critical and economical practice of medicine. I suspect that the students taught to approach diagnosis as a process of further information collection become the young doctors who develop the approach of the diagnostic work-up and so the costs increase and play their part in causing the medicopolitical trouble affecting most countries. I believe that a more scientific approach could improve matters by the wiser use of technology. But, back to diagnosis.

I suspect the student perceives the clinician as employing a careful system of collecting information and having instant access to a large store of knowledge. When the information he collects from a patient is fed into the store, the diagnosis is revealed. In other words, the diagnostic process is inductive.

The Popperian view of science is that it is not inductive but hypothetico-deductive. In brief, I want to argue that we should recognize that the diagnostic process is similar, and that in our teaching we should encourage the habit of generating hypotheses more than we do.

Let me remind you of the studies of the Leeds group in which they compared the performance of house surgeons with consultants and registrars as diagnosticians (9). These show that the more experienced clinicians conducted shorter interviews, adapted their questioning to the patient's problem and used questions with a greater 'utility' – i.e. questions which are more likely to contribute to the solution of the problem.

I suggest we can draw two inferences from these studies: first, the more experienced clinicians are thinking of possibilities and this is why they conduct the interview in the way they do; secondly, the change in performance between the junior and senior clinicians does not just reflect a difference of ability or experience but a change of mental habits or processes. And I think we should be able to encourage the acquisition of these habits and processes sooner than seven or eight years after starting medical school.

What are these mental habits – what is the diagnostic process? I do not think we really know. It may be partly logical reasoning, partly an assessment of probabilities, partly pattern recognition (10). At present I think we must accept all of these as being used to some extent by all or most doctors. But I believe that, whichever is true, they all lead to the early generation of hypotheses and their critical examination rather than to information gleaning.

I would like to pursue this idea further, using as my model the general medical consultation. I could be criticized on the grounds that little of medicine, particularly in primary care or general practice, is like a general medical consultation but I would defend myself on two grounds. First, the general medical consultation is a discipline which all doctors must become familiar with and which for most students in most medical schools provides their introduction to the practice of medicine. Secondly, the difference between this consultation and other clinical contacts is not as great as students and general practitioners commonly think if the mental activities I am going to try to describe are admitted by teachers and encouraged in students.

Some Assertions. I shall begin with two assertions about the way we think – not just when faced with diagnostic problems but when faced with almost anything we have to interpret.

1. We cannot passively observe. Ideas (hypotheses) 'spring to mind' at the first hint or clue. We then examine the information our senses provide for support or rejection of the hypotheses in an active searching way.

2. We can actively entertain only a limited number of possibilities at the one time.

Let me expand.

I have already mentioned Popper's strong case that the scientist thinks of possibilities. There is good evidence that this is true of simpler matters like vision (11, 12). In fact, Gregory (11) explicitly compares visual perception with science and argues that perceptions are hypotheses.

My second assertion arises as a question implicitly posed by the first. If we approach problems by trying out possible solutions, how many possible solutions can we try at one time? In the clinical context, how many possibilities can we have in mind when listening to the patient's answer to one of our questions and in prompting us to think of the next question?

Obviously we are able to think of more than one, and in fact we would be very bad at solving any problems if we could only think of one solution at a time. But I doubt that the number is very large. For fairly simple matters Miller (13) has suggested that the number is about seven. For more complex matters such as diagnostic possibilities I think the number is probably between three and five. Let me take four.

So, in a nutshell, I am suggesting that the experienced clinician thinks of possibilities from the earliest clue and the number he thinks of can be no more than four. Early moves in the interview are directed to arrange the possibilities to fit in with this contraint.

I would cite a number of studies in recent years whose findings support this assertion (14, 15, 16).

Let me immediately emphasize that the list of four possibilities is not the same as a differential diagnosis. It may include procedural categories such as 'if it isn't (a) or (b) then I must "watch and wait", "refer for specialist opinion" or "do such and such a test" '.

Some Qualifications and Expansions. There are occasions when we flounder and find it difficult or impossible either to set up hypotheses or to formulate them in a way which we feel will embrace the solution of the problem. When this happens we resign ourselves to taking a full history and making a complete examination 'with an open mind'. Sometimes we ask for a second opinion, not, I submit, because of the limitation of our knowledge or technique but because a 'fresh mind' is needed.

Because he is limited in the amount of information he can carry and the possibilities he can entertain, the clinician tends to code 'bits' of information into 'chunks'. Thus if he thinks of the possibility of iron deficiency he may quickly look at the nails, the mucous membranes and the tongue and enquire about blood loss so that he can code all these 'bits' into the single, more useful and less demanding 'chunk'. Other examples would be fever, shock, heart failure, hyperthyroidism.

In addition to solving the diagnostic problem, the doctor of course uses the interview to establish a relationship and to assess the sort of person the patient is, so that his management will not simply be that described in textbooks for the diagnosed condition but will also be appropriate for the particular patient. This is where I would be prepared to accept medicine can legitimately be said to be an art.

The Generation of the Initial Hypothesis. This is the central diagnostic skill. If, as I have asserted, the doctor can think of only four possibilities at once, how does he order his mind?

Although he may be alerted to certain possibilities from the very beginning, he usually keeps his mind as passive as possible ('in neutral') until he has identified certain charactertistics of the problem: the history and features of the patient's complaint. Usually his enquiry does not get far before his mind goes 'into gear' and puts up its list of hypotheses.

Seeing the age and sex of the patient, the clinician is unlikely to go beyond the duration of the complaint (and, in the case of pain, the approximate site) before he has his list. The list can be no greater than four and will be a mixture of diagnostic and procedural possibilities weighted both by probability and importance. Sometimes the list can be very simple: 'either (a) or something else'. Thus, for example, central chest pain in middle age – 'myocardial ischaemia or something else'; a lump in the breast – 'carcinoma or something else'.

To generalize, I would call the initial strategy 'three plus one', by which I mean that the clinician will seek to develop a list which can be no more complicated than 'either (a), (b), (c) or something else'. I think this is what Kozielecki (17) means by the 'catch all' strategy.

What does the clinician do when the hypotheses leap into his mind? He does not like to leave the patient's complaint until he has reduced the list to 'three plus one' and he will ask questions designed to rearrange the list. Skill and experience lead him to select powerful questions, i.e. questions which are easy to answer and which will refute or reduce the probability of some of the hypotheses. Sometimes he will use questions which are powerful in a positive sense – the answers greatly increase the probability of a hypothesis he already has thought of. But I think a good clinician, like a good scientist, prefers the former at this stage. It must be emphasized that the care, aggressiveness, persistence with which the clinician asks these questions are dependent on the possibilities he already has in mind. The most careful recording of the history by questionnaire or objective interviewer does not compare with the seasoned clinician in this activity for two reasons, one fundamental and one practical. First, the passive observer cannot register significant information if his mind has no use for it at the time it is obtained. Secondly, the signal/noise ratio of most clinical information is low unless it is actively processed by directed senses.

I am not going into the subsequent clinical procedure in any systematic way, but I would like to make a few relevant if unconnected points.

What is the place of routine questioning? I think much lower than students are led to believe and on the whole directed to other objectives than solving the diagnostic problem, such as screening for other conditions, developing baseline information or finding out more about the patient's background.

I thought I would compile a list of routine questions from general physicians. I tried to find out what questions they feel obliged to ask in addition to those required to solve the presenting problem. It seems the number is somewhere between 15 and 20 but fewer than 10 of them are common to all the physicians I studied. I am not going to reveal these questions because the list elicits such argument and scorn and distracts people from my main point.

Next, what about physical examination? The seasoned clinician rarely does a routine physical examination. That remark does not mean that he goes about the physical examination devoid of any routine; it means that in a routine sequence he specifically seeks bits or chunks of information with a concentration that stems from the short list of possibilities he has already in mind. The physical examination is of course generally accepted as not being as important as the history in refining the list of diagnostic possibilities and the diagnosis is radically changed by the examination in only about 10 per cent of consultations (18). And I suspect that 9 of these 10 per cent depend on findings elicited in a minute or so.

Now I must correct the impression I may well have given that we should not teach students to take a full history or do a thorough physical examination. I must hasten to insist that we do not abandon that goal. What I suggest is that, having achieved it, we then do not move on to the next step. Having inculcated the repertoire of subroutines, we do not teach the students flexibility in the employment of the subroutines in the examination of the possible solutions. We do not encourage him to think of possibilities and adapt his procedures to them. Or, rather, if we do attempt to do this, then the studies of Leaper et al. (9) show that we are not very successful. Popper would probably suggest that we are much better at filling the buckets of our students' minds than in training their searchlights.

What do the Books Teach? I have examined all the popular books on diagnostic techniques written in English. I think it fair to say that, with one or two exceptions, they emphasize the care and accuracy of information garnering as a preliminary to the creation of a list of possibilities. Some of the books recognize that their prescriptions do not accord with what the experienced clinician does. They more or less say 'with experience he will learn short cuts'. I avow that this view and teaching are fundamentally wrong. The experienced clinician in a hurry is not pursuing short cuts through an information-gleaning system; he is doing what he does all the time – thinking of possibilities and adapting his procedure to those possibilities. When under pressure, he admits to this sort of behaviour because he has to. Nevertheless, it is really what he does all the time. Just as Medawar suggested that the scientific paper may be a hoax in that, whatever its value as a means of sharing information, it does not reflect the scientific process, so I would like to suggest that the case record we traditionally require is a hoax in that, whatever its value in conveying clinical information, it does not represent the approach of the seasoned clinician.

Implications for Teaching. So far I have not developed any prescriptions for changes in teaching following from the views expressed above, but I do not think such prescriptions would need to be very difficult or that they would conflict with much that goes on today. Perhaps there should be some return to a closer intimacy in the apprenticeship relationship such that the student is admitted to the intimacy of his teacher's mind in real situations rather than just in formal teaching situations. Perhaps we could also invent some 'games' which encourage the development of economical diagnostic strategies.

Having been a subject, I am impressed with the potential of Dr Howard Barrows' programmed or simulated patients as a medium for such games. They are particularly valuable because they permit 'stop – why? – start again' type teaching in acute medical situations. These are just the situations in which the hypothetico-deductive approach to problems is unavoidable and in which procedural hypotheses may take precedence over diagnostic ones. And, of course, for all sorts of reasons, in most schools the student is rarely more than an observer of the handling of such problems. Unfortunately, while most neurological physical signs can be simulated, the same is not true of affection of other systems.

Before closing, one must face the question whether the acquisition of the mental habits of the seasoned clinician is an important matter. After all, the students get there in the end when they are housemen. But I think it does matter very much indeed for two reasons: first, most hospital medicine is done by house officers and therefore patterns of practice and expense are dictated by their habits; secondly, for many of these trainees the next step is general practice where most of the problems do not demand nor time permit the routines they have acquired.

Unfortunately, in most teaching hospitals the layers of staff, gamesmanship, status, and so on promote the mindless work-up. There are also forces at work in society which make it easier to do things than not to do them – so-called defensive medicine. All of us, from the junior student to the senior teacher, could help by asking more often 'what's in your mind?'

Let me finish by giving the last word to Medawar, a very perceptive non-clinical scientist.

> 'In commencement addresses and other uplifting declarations, clinicians who discourse on the "spirit of medicine", will always point out that, while there is a large and profoundly important scientific element in the practice of medicine, there is also an indefinable artistry, an imaginative insight, and medicine (they will tell us) is born of a marriage between the two. But then (it seems to me) the speaker spoils everything by getting the bride and groom confused. It is the unbiased observation, the apparatus, the ritual of fact finding and the inductive mumbo jumbo that the clinician thinks of as "scientific", and the other element, intuitive and logically unscripted which he thinks of as a creative art.' (19).

References

1. Campbell, E.J.M. (1976a). *Lancet,* **i**, 134.
2. Campbell, E.J.M. (1976b). *Clinical Science,* **51**, 1.

3. Magee, B. (1973). *Popper.* London, Fontana.
4. Porter, R. and Birch, J. (1971). *Identification of Asthma,* Ciba Foundation Study Group No. 38. Edinburgh and London, Churchill Livingstone.
5. Scadding, J.G. (1967). *Lancet,* **ii**, 877.
6. Wulff, H. (1976). *Rational Diagnosis and Treatment.* Oxford, Blackwell.
7. Kuhn, T.S. (1970). *The Structure of Scientific Revolutions,* 2nd edn. Chicago and London, University of Chicago.
8. Dudley, H.A.F. (1976). *Medical Hypotheses,* **2**, 164.
9. Leaper, D.J., Gill, P.W., Staniland, J.R., Horrocks, J.C. and de Dombal, F.T. (1973). *British Medical Journal,* **3**, 569.
10. Card, W.I. and Good, I.J. (1971). *British Medical Journal,* **1**, 718.
11. Abercrombie, M.L.J. (1960). *The Anatomy of Judgement.* Harmondsworth, Middx., Penguin.
12. Gregory, R.L. 1973). *Proceedings of the Royal Institution,* **46**, 117.
13. Miller, G.A. (1956). *Psychological Reviews,* **63**, 81.
14. Barrows, H.S. and Bennett, K. (1972). *Archives of Neurology,* **26**, 273.
15. Elstein, A.S., Kogan, N., Shulman, I.S., Jason, H. and Loupe, M.U. (1972). *Journal of Medical Education,* **47**, 85.
16. Neufeld, V., Morma, G., Feightner, J. and Barrows, H.S. (1975). *Proceedings of 14th Annual Conference on Research in Medical Education,* p. 149. Washington DC, Assoc. of Medical Colleges.
17. Kozielecki, J. (1972). *Acta Psychologica,* **36**, 370.
18. Hampton, J.R., Harrison, M.J.G., Mitchell, J.R.A., Prichard, J.S. and Seymour, C. (1975). *British Medical Journal,* **2**, 486.
19. Medawar, P.B. (1969). *Induction and Intuition in Scientific Thought.* London, Methuen.

11

Algorithmic, Sequential/Logical Approaches to Clinical Management

H.A.F. Dudley

Both Professor Card and Professor Moran Campbell have dealt with the methods by which doctors attempt to reach decisions about patients. Though our lack of knowledge makes any description incomplete, and there is clearly much room for further investigation, it seems that we may use a combination of Popperian hypothesis-deduction (1, 2) and Bayesian induction by which to test our provisional ideas in order to heighten the probability of a correct choice. Some philosophers, and particularly those who follow Hume, would hold that this is an unholy alliance but clearly, within our restricted universe of medical events, it works. We begin the medical encounter with an ill-formulated hypothesis which the accumulation of facts may support or confute. The weight of the evidence is assessed in probabilistic or likelihood terms and eventually a threshold is reached on which some action is based. A new sequence may then be triggered and the same process pursued aimed now, not at the question 'what is wrong?', but at the proposition 'what should be done?' (3).

This form of logic is often sequential in two respects: first, as Campbell has emphasized, Miller's rule operates – we are unable to deal with more than a few facts or concepts at any one time; secondly, it often takes time to observe the outcome of a decision or to make a further observation or test. Thus, the decision-making process lends itself to expression in flow chart terms, a technique which has been widely used by a number of authors, including myself. Influenced by the binary logic of the computer world (and perhaps, though less clearly, of the real world as well) these charts or logic trees tend to be drawn up on YES/NO, GO/NO GO terms. Obviously each node in such a tree can be as macro or as micro as one wishes, by which I mean containing more or less of a weighted sum of the available and relevant evidence. It may also be at a low or high conceptual level, much as are computer languages. In practice all such nodes are

Bayesian and, as I have pointed out before, this is true even of an electronic OR gate, even though here the probability of things going the opposite way from expected, when a particular signal is applied, is vanishingly small.

If medical process can be *expressed* in this way – and in doing so we do not need to assume that this is the *pattern* of practice – then it is now only a short step towards trying to organize a flow chart in such a way that only a minimum number of nodes are traversed to reach a terminal decision, or more generally to carry an individual from problem to solution. At the same time, at each node we shall wish to collect evidence which will provide the greatest discriminant value between the choice of the two exit pathways from it. To adopt such a strategy is to be parsimonious and determinant at the same time. It does also mean that the quality of a manoeuvre, in terms of its effect on the patient, is initially neglected. For example, I can nearly always make the diagnosis of intra-abdominal malignancy by a wide laparotomy and therefore the most parsimonious and determinant pathway would be to say that if abdominal malignancy is suspected, laparotomy should be performed. However, this neglects the fact that laparotomy is dangerous and painful for the patient and that it is costly (in money and resources, that is) to the community.

We need then some calculus which will permit us to construct sequential processes for decision making which have the following characteristics:

1. Clear-cut objectives given a particular problem, e.g. whether or not to open the abdomen if a patient presents with acute abdominal pain.
2. A minimal path strategy in terms of the number of nodes traversed.
3. The use of minimal and discriminant data at each node.
4. A cost analysis for the patient and for society of the whole system and for each node within the system.

Unfortunately, no such calculus exists in medicine. Attempts to build systems must therefore be empirical. Over the years a number of workers have done just this with interesting results which can be basically summarized as indicating that most diagnostic goals can be reached by pathways which are trivially short. To quote but a few examples, jaundice can be discriminated as to cause with a considerable degree of accuracy by the Bayesian analysis only of the data present on history examination and early laboratory tests (4). In a number of surgical situations, either of diagnosis or management, it is possible to provide simple answers to relatively complex questions with considerable speed. For example, the need to order a chest x-ray preoperatively (Fig. 11.1) or whether to manage a patient conservatively after acute upper gastrointestinal haemorrhage (Fig. 11.2).

Though we do not have a formal calculus, it is clear that the wealth of information stored in the mind of a clinician provides a useful starting point for the development of a semi-formal decision chart. I can best illustrate this by referring to my own experience of cancer of the breast.

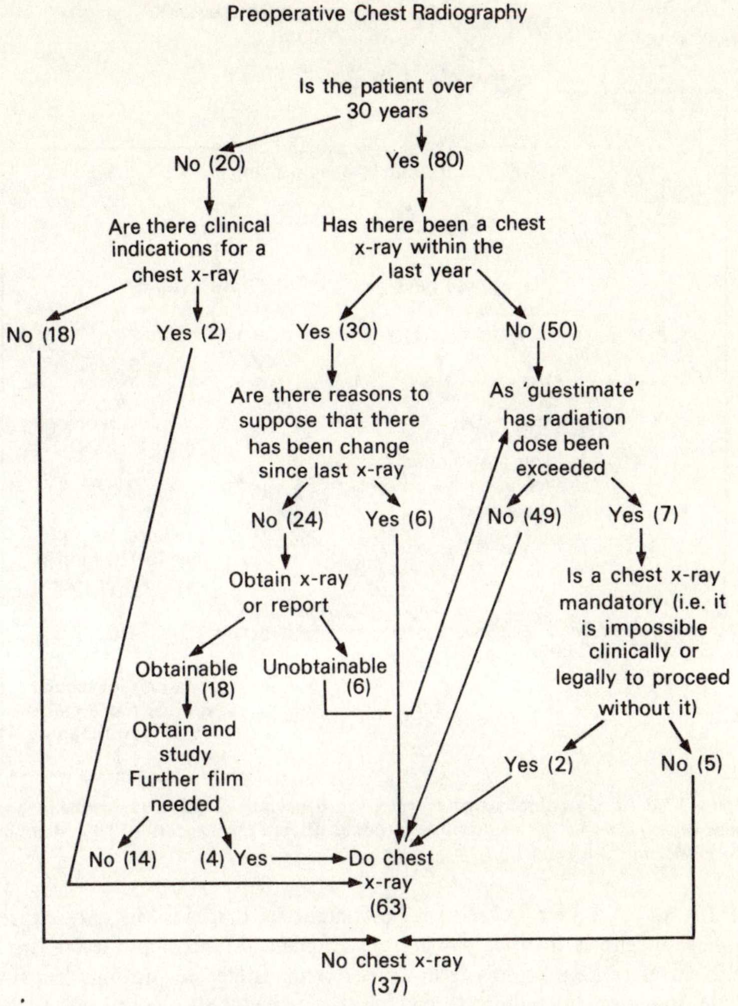

Figure 11.1 An algorithmic approach to ordering a chest x-ray in the patient who is to undergo non-cardiopulmonary surgery. The figures are a theoretical analysis of possible savings. (Based on the data of Rees et al. (5).)

The *problem* is to resolve the issue – is a given lump cancer or not – with a minimum expenditure of time and effort and a minimum of cost in the terms I have already defined. The *process* involved is the translation of a statement in one frame to that in another (3). In this instance, transfer is from a clinical to a histopathological diagnosis of malignancy. Along the way we need to gather data, which may be determinantly useful in subsequent management of the patient, about the extent and dissemination

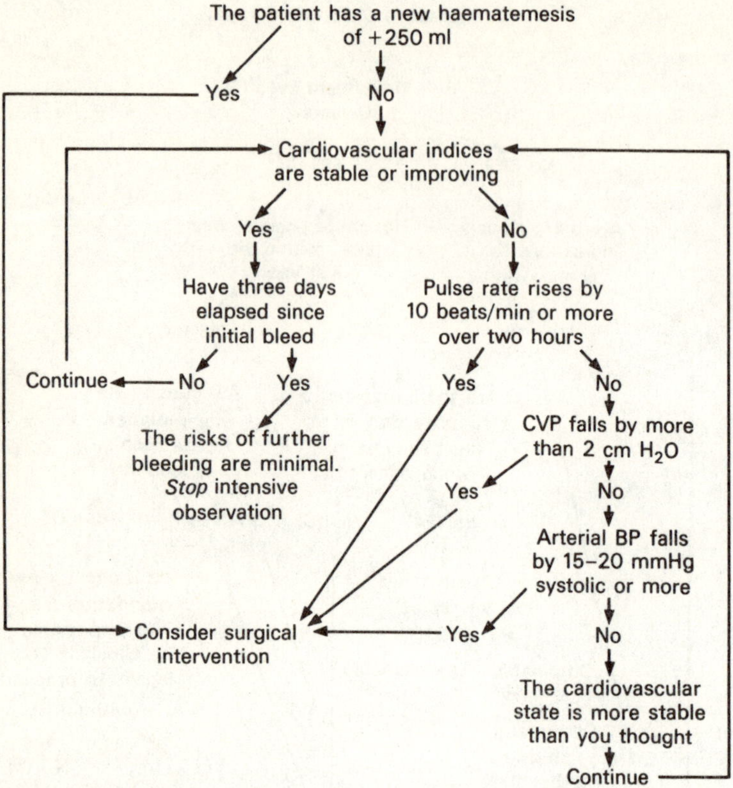

Figure 11.2 An algorithm, based on observed behaviour of patients, for the management of acute upper gastrointestinal bleeding. (Based on the data of Northfield and Smith (6), and Dudley (3).)

of the disease. Our experience has taught us that we can only express clinical diagnosis in three categories – benign, doubtful and malignant – with an error rate of less than 10 per cent. Thereafter nothing less than some statement in cellular terms – cyto- or histopathological will suffice to provide the basis for action. Thus, the diagnostic pathway inevitably leads to fine needle aspiration for cytopathology and from there to some form of histopathological biopsy (using drill or specifically designed needle such as the Trucut). A flow chart can be constructed with these objectives in mind against a background of (a) accuracy of the techniques, (b) logistic gains or losses, (c) patient gains or losses. We are at present using this technique to analyse losses and gains for patients who present with breast lumps, but both our own evidence (8) and that of Professor Hughes' group (9) suggest significant gains for the patient and in logistics.

The foregoing is an exercise in sequential and economical diagnosis. Essex's techniques for clinical diagnosis in a developing country are similar (10). However, sequential methods are not the only way that discrimination may be sought. De Dombal (11) and Gunn (12) have both shown how the use of Bayesian techniques to process at one moment the information derived from a structured history and physical examination can save unnecessary surgical operations and fruitless admissions in patients who present with acute abdominal pain. Here the analysis is terminal – that is the data is collected and analysed as a whole by probability summation to give diagnostic probabilities which can guide the clinician. These approaches aim, as do sequential methods, to select the most discriminant items of the clinical record and to sum these and these alone – clearly again a parsimonious approach.

Both the examples I have given are highly organized to deal with repetitive situations – the breast lump or the patient with acute abdominal pain. The same general strategy can be applied *ad hoc* if one reflects on a few simple principles that I have outlined. First, what is the frame in which diagnosis or merely data must be organized and expressed so that action can be taken? Is it clinical, as in the decision to operate upon the patient with an acute abdomen? Is it endoscopic, as in the decision to manage an instance of acute bleeding from the upper gastrointestinal tract? Is it physiological, as in the demonstration of acute arterial hypoxia in a postoperative patient? Is it pathological, as in the example of a breast lump or, say, a young man with firm rubbery glands in one side of the neck? Second, what is the shortest path by which diagnosis in a chosen frame can be reached? Third, does this pathway carry any obvious gains or, more particularly, losses for the patient? An *ad hoc* calculus of this kind alters many of our clinical attitudes. To mention but a few, it introduces laparoscopy to the clinical diagnosis of acute abdominal pain so saving beds, unnecessary scars and possible complications (13). It can shorten the investigation period for patients with jaundice and gall bladder disease; it concentrates attention on the choice of a liver scintiscan or ultrasound for the initial investigation of patients in the cancer age group who have vague abdominal symptoms and a palpable liver. In general, it suggests that we should look with a critical eye at the long lists of investigations for which those of us who are older (if not much wiser) blame on our junior staff.

Investigative medicine has tended to be cumulative rather than selective – any new test is added on rather than an examination made for its ability to substitute for the old. Often it is evaluated in isolation for its diagnostic or procedural worth so that when it is said that (say) it is 90 per cent effective, this figure is not placed in any perspective of what was achieved by previous techniques and at what cost. A good current example is endoscopic retrograde cholangiopancreatography (ERCP). This is a highly effective diagnostic tool in the elucidation of jaundice, but as far as I am aware its place in decision making as distinct from anatomical diagnosis vis-à-vis other investigations has not been established. Recently, in a gush of enthusiasm, a medical editor described as a 'dream paper' (14) a comparison of the ability of ERCP and percutaneous hepatic cholangiography (PHC) to 'diagnose' jaundice – a comparison that favoured ERCP in pathological terms (15). However, this paper singularly failed to tell us at any point how decision making had been or could be influenced. Both investigations might be classified as sufficient – with the edge on ERCP as the primary procedure provided that costs and complexity were discounted – but neither was established as necessary. More precisely, neither was defined in terms of *when* it was necessary in individual patients. I do not wish to chastise investigative work of this kind – it is necessary to identify the limits of a technique by using it on a defined population. However, this of itself is not enough and the results of investigating any diagnostic or procedural 'advance' must form the component of a subsequent analysis of the *real* place in practical medicine of proposed changes. It is possible, but by no means established, that some of the theoretical models which have been proposed (see, for example, References 3, 16, 17; Chapters 10 and 12 in this volume) may provide the background for the statement of useful theorems even though they are only facets of a total and confused reality of medical procedure.

Finally, let me turn to real life and cost effectiveness. In the UK, though we have talked about the matter, we have rarely taken useful action to bring it about. Some pioneer radiological studies can tell us a good deal about what might be done: for example, intravenous pyelography is singularly lacking in cost effectiveness in the investigation of hypertension (18) and, as I have mentioned, blanket preoperative chest x-rays are also very wasteful; the place of mammography in breast disease either as a screening process or for diagnosis of an established state is also unknown though under intensive study. And yet we exercise hardly any control over these matters in our day-to-day care. As a surgical colleague remarked the other day, 'Any casualty officer or houseman can order any x-ray he thinks is warranted on any patient without let or hindrance at immense cost; by contrast, if I want a new instrument, which I know to be necessary for my work, it has to go through a number of committees and may then be refused'.

Now I do not suggest that we should start to organize elaborate peer reviews or complex audits. I believe neither has proved its worth as instruments for assessing and influencing behaviour (19). Recent evidence from the USA supports this view, at least for surgery (20). Utilization review and peer-directed audit are extremely costly and singularly without influence on the behaviour of individuals. Rather I am proposing that we use the principle of parsimony (Chapter 12, this volume) to examine our common clinical manoeuvres, both investigative and in terms of management, so as to ascertain if we are using, first, the most economical medical logic and, second, ways of procedure which are cost effective. If some agreement can be reached in terms of what should be done, then there is a structural basis for analysing departures from this norm in ways which are meaningful in clinical medical terms rather than primarily in the language of economics. We are a long way from this goal, but progress is being made along the road in a number of centres.

References

1. Medawar, P.D. (1969). *Induction and Intuition in Scientific Thought.* London, Methuen.
2. Dudley, H. (1970). The clinical task. *Lancet,* **ii,** 1352-1354.
3. Dudley, H. (1976). Clinical method is all wrong. *Medical Hypotheses,* **2,** 164-167.
4. Stern, R.B., Knill-Jones, R.P. and Williams, R. (1975). Use of a computer program for diagnosing jaundice in district hospitals and specialised liver unit. *British Medical Journal,* **2,** 659-662.
5. Rees, A.M., Roberts, C.J., Bligh, A.S. and Evans, K.T. (1976). Routine pre-operative chest radiography in non-cardiopulmonary surgery. *British Medical Journal,* **1,** 1333-1336.
6. Northfield, T.C. and Smith, T. (1970). Central venous pressure in clinical management of acute gastrointestinal bleeding. *Lancet,* **ii,** 584-586.
7. Dudley, H. (1977). In: *Hamilton Bailey's Emergency Surgery,* 10th edn. Ed. by H. Dudley. Bristol, John Wright.
8. Dudley, H. (1975). Clinical algorithms. In: *Advanced Medical Systems: Issues and Challenges,* pp. 191-200. Ed. by Charles D. Flagle. From 6th Annual Meeting of the Society for Advanced Medical Systems (SAMS), Baltimore, Maryland. New York, Stratton Intercontinental Medical Book Corp.
9. Roberts, J.G., Preece, P.E., Bolton, P.M., Baum, M. and Hughes, L.E. (1975). The 'tru-cut' biopsy in breast cancer. *Clinical Oncology,* **1,** 297-303.
10. Essex, B.J. (1975). Approach to rapid problem solving in clinical medicine. *British Medical Journal,* **2,** 34-36.
11. de Dombal, F.T. (1973). Surgical diagnosis assisted by a computer. *Proceedings of the Royal Society* series B, **184,** 433-440.
12. Gunn, A.A. (1976). The diagnosis of acute abdominal pain with computer analysis. *Journal of the Royal College of Surgeons Edinburgh,* **21,** 170-172.
13. Sugarbacker, P.H., Bloom, B.S., Sanders, J.H. and Wilson, R.E. (1975). Pre-operative laparoscopy in diagnosis of acute abdominal pain. *Lancet,* **i,** 442-445.
14. Conn, H.O., Redeker, A.G. and Zimmon, D.S. (1976). PTC versus ERC – an editor's dream. *Gastroenterology,* **71,** 520-521.
15. Elias, E., Hamlyn, A.N., Jain, S., Long, R.G., Summerfield, J.A., Dick, R. and Sherlock, S. (1976). A randomized trial of percutaneous transhepatic cholangiography with the Chiba needle versus endoscopic retrograde cholangiography for bile duct visualization in jaundice. *Gastroenterology,* **71,** 439-443.
16. Elstein, A.S., Kagan, N., Shulman, L.S., Jason, H. and Loupe, M.J. (1972). Methods and theories in the study of medical enquiry. *Journal of Medical Education,* **47,** 85-92.
17. Elstein, A.S. (1976). Clinical judgement: psychological research and medical practice. *Science,* **194,** 696-700.
18. Kreel, L., Elton, A., Habershon, R., Mason, A.M.S. and Meade, T.N. (1974). Use of intravenous urography. *British Medical Journal,* **4,** 31-33.
19. Dudley, H. (1974). Necessity of surgical audit. *British Medical Journal,* **1,** 275-277.
20. McSherry, C.K. (1976). Quality assurance: the cost of utilisation review and the educational value of medical audit in a university hospital. *Surgery,* **80,** 122-129.

12

Parsimony in Clinical Medicine

Wilfrid Card

Since Hippocrates, the doctor has made observations on patients and decisions about them. These decisions are based on the doctor's training and subsequent experience and he may be said to arrive at them privately. It is now possible to envisage a formal system of medicine in which many, and ultimately perhaps all, decisions can be calculated and in this sense made public. This possibility exists because of the development of relevant mathematical disciplines, probablity and decision theory, while the computer makes calculations possible which were previously unthinkable.

In this formal system, the doctor can be thought of as moving through a decision tree making a sequence of decisions. Such a tree is symbolized in Fig. 12.1 and the decision maker moves on a path from left to right.

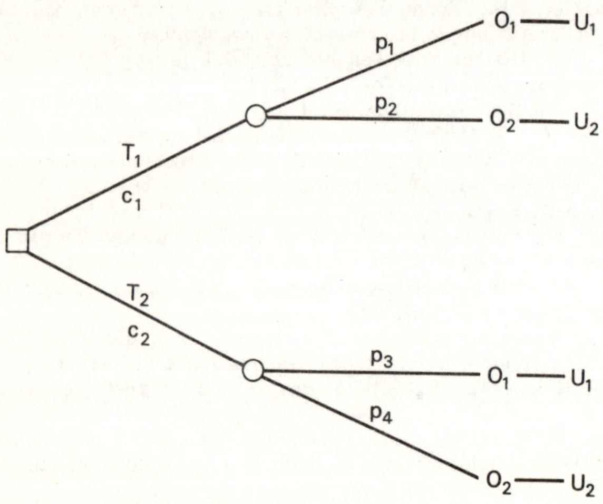

Figure 12.1 Decision tree with two treatments and two outcomes

The decision tree contains two kinds of nodes which alternate: square nodes where a decision is taken and round nodes which represent the result of the decision. While the decision is under the complete control of the doctor, the result of the decision cannot be foreseen with certainty, and the node is said to be a random node, the result occurring with a certain probability only. With the knowledge thus gained the doctor may now make a further decision and thus move through the tree.

A simple decision would be a choice between two treatments (Fig. 12.1), T_1 and T_2, where a null treatment is mathematically considered to be a treatment. Suppose the patient is a young man who has had a small haematemesis. There is no previous history of chronic ulceration but there is a history of taking aspirin and the decision is whether or not to move him to hospital for blood transfusion. To analyse such a decision, it is necessary to know the set of treatments; the outcomes of each treatment, e.g. bleeding recurs, bleeding does not recur; the probabilities of each outcome, conditional on the state of the patient and the particular treatment (p_1, p_2, p_3, p_4); and it is also necessary to have a number, thought of as a measure of value or worth, to be attached to each outcome. This number will be called a utility (U_1, U_2). It is now possible to set out the expected value or utility of each treatment, where by 'expected' is meant its value on the average.

The expected value of a treatment is the sum of the expected values of the outcomes less the cost (c_1, c_2) of that treatment, or, in symbols:

$$\in.U(T_1) = p_1U_1 + p_2U_2 - c_1$$

...1

$$\in.U(T_2) = p_3U_1 + p_4U_2 - c_2$$

'Cost' we may think of as a kind of negative utility and the concept has to include the actual monetary cost and also what may be called the 'biological' cost to the patient, that is, any pain or disturbance caused by the treatment and any danger to life. With these expressions, we can now, in principle, calculate the best treatment as the one which has the greatest expected utility.

In mathematics the expression of a problem in defined form is often half the battle, while the other half is the problem of estimation, in this situation of utilities, of probabilities of outcomes, and of costs.

The general problem of the estimation of the utilities of outcomes, that is, of those states of health which arise from the treatment, is unsolved (1, 2) but some progress has been made in a simple system using a wagering technique (3). This technique was suggested in the earliest writings on decision theory (4).

We imagine three states of health, S_1, S_2 and S_3, such that S_3 is preferable to S_2 and S_2 is preferable to S_1. This is equivalent to saying that the utility of S_3, $U(S_3)$, is greater than the utility of S_2, $U(S_2)$, and that the utility of S_2, $U(S_2)$, is greater than the utility of S_1, $U(S_1)$. We then imagine that the patient is in the middle state, S_2, and there is some treatment which gives him a chance of moving into the state S_3 with probability p, and therefore a probability, 1–p, of moving into the less preferable state, S_1. If the probability p were 1, that is, if it were absolutely certain that the patient would move into the preferred state, he would choose the treatment without question. Similarly, if the chance of improvement were nil, that is, p = 0, and he were certain to become worse, the patient would never accept the treatment. It is therefore argued that there must be an intermediate value of p at which the patient would be indifferent to moving from the state S_2. At this point of indifference,

$$U(S_2) = p.U(S_3) + (1-p)\,U(S_1) \qquad ...2$$

If therefore we know the utilities of S_3 and S_1, or assign arbitrary values to them, we can calculate the utility of the intermediate state, S_2.

This estimation becomes easier if it is possible to have a set of states of health which differ in only one variable, such as a change in visual acuity, so that the states of health can be represented along one dimension. In such a set a number of wagers becomes possible. The patient situation can be simulated and be presented to a number of subjects for their estimates of the probability of each wager, one that they would themselves advise. From such a set of wagers, utility estimates can be made corresponding to each state of health and plotted against the corresponding visual acuity. Using this technique, Card and his colleagues (3) showed that in eight subjects whom they tested, the utility function was linear against the logarithm of the visual acuity. By 'function' is meant a rule whereby a utility value can be assigned to any particular measure of visual acuity; geometrically it will plot as a straight line (Fig. 12.2). From this linear

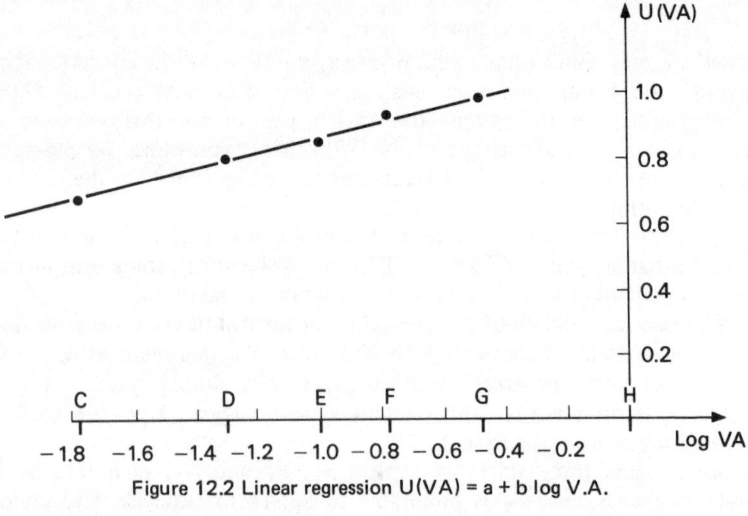

Figure 12.2 Linear regression U(VA) = a + b log V.A.

relationship follows the somewhat surprising result that the minimal odds for success against failure that any surgeon would demand before agreeing to operate in any of the simulated situations would be the same for all surgeons and would be independent of their actual utility functions.

The above is an example of the utility function of a set of unidimensional states of health but of course the states of health which are commonly encountered are multidimensional. The problem here is much more complex and the first step might be to decide the dimensions along which such states might be measured. It would be preferable to keep these as few as possible; danger to life, severity and duration of symptoms, and degree of disability for work and recreation are three dimensions which might suffice. But we are faced with a further difficulty.

Equation 1 indicates that the costs of the treatment stand to be subtracted from the expected gain of the treatment, any gain being an improvement in the state of health. If this subtraction is to be made, the costs of treatment must be measured in the same units as the gain in utility. Now the costs can be thought of as partly monetary, and a cost accountant could make some estimate of the monetary cost of treatment, but they are also what may be termed biological, that is, they may include symptoms such as pain or even danger to life. If the utilities and costs are to be measured in the same units, it is convenient to find a monetary equivalent to a utility, and this implies measuring the monetary value of a state of health, that is, of a human life.

This need to produce a monetary equivalent to a human life produces considerable resistance in the minds of many doctors and laymen but this seems to be due to a misunderstanding. In a country such as the UK, the National Health Service has limited resources and has to deploy these to the best advantage and no one has yet suggested a more rational way than by the use of decision theory. The monetary value of a human life is thus a notional value and it bears no relation to the value an individual would place on the life of a member of his own family which he might well describe as priceless.

Economists looking on a human being as a wealth producing and wealth consuming unit, have produced a figure for the value of an average life at different ages, discounting future production and future consumption (5, 6, 7). However, society does not only look on the individual in this way but, when he is no longer capable of work, provides him with some retirement pension and various social goods such as access to parks, free libraries, etc., thus demonstrating its valuation of him as a human being. This valuation stands to be added to the figure obtained by regarding him purely as an economic unit.

The above analysis has omitted any discussion on the estimation of the probability of an outcome given the treatment, that is, the prognosis. The allocation to a prognostic class is mathematically very similar to the allocation of a patient to a disease class, and both will be discussed below. The example above of the choice of treatments of a symptom could of course become sequential if the bleeding recurred. The fact of recurrence itself is evidence that alters the probabilities of outcomes and therefore the expected utilities of different treatments. But usually we do not treat a single symptom by itself but the patient has a whole series of complaints and we have first to diagnose them and then allot a specific treatment. By discussing the decision on treatment first we emphasize its importance and that the process of diagnosis, though antecedent in time, is secondary to it.

It is first necessary to consider the meaning and use of the word 'diagnosis'. The literal meaning is 'thorough knowledge' (8) but this, as Cohen says, is represented for convenience by a diagnostic 'label'. In the sense of 'thorough knowledge', the statement, 'this patient with a chronic duodenal ulcer will do well if treated surgically' is a diagnosis, though it contains, besides a disease label, a prognosis based on treatment. 'Diagnosis' is often used in a restricted sense of applying disease labels and, in this sense, can be thought of as 'provisional formulae designed for action' (9). In either case we use a disease label and it is necessary to consider what we mean by a disease and why in any formal system of medicine this concept is found to be necessary.

A disease is an abstraction derived from the study of a number of sick people and not a 'morbid entity' in the sense of Sydenham, hence the aphorism 'Diseases do not exist; only sick people'. Sometimes the disease has a definite cause (for example, typhoid fever) and it then becomes possible to provide a single logical definition of the disease in terms of its aetiology, for example, of a positive blood culture in the first week of the disease. Clearly not all diseases are capable of definition in this way and the definition may have to be a statistical one in terms of a number of attributes. This problem is not confined to medicine but occurs wherever a class, for example, a biological species or an archaeological period such as the early Bronze Age, is defined statistically in terms of a number of attributes. If we think of each medical attribute or indicant as occurring on a dimension in a hyperspace, then the individual appears as a point in this space and the 'disease' will appear as a cloud of points representing individuals suffering from that disease, roughly separable from another cloud of points representing another 'disease'. Mathematical techniques exist, such as cluster analysis, to detect such clusters and thus to give some definition of a disease which has no single defining logical characteristic (10).

Why do we need to introduce this concept of disease? The mathematician may ask why we cannot describe the patient as a set of indicants, technically a vector, and from this, by some decision function, arrive at a specific treatment. We should thus jump straight from the symptoms, signs and all the laboratory findings to a treatment, avoiding the intermediate step of allocation to a disease class. The answer seems to be that the size of the patient vector and the number of potential treatments make this impossible. However, it becomes possible when we have narrowed down the number of treatments and can deal with a manageable set of indicants and this has been exemplified in the treatment of depression (11). Should we 'diagnose' the depressive state further by allocating the patient to the class of either 'endogenous' or 'reactive' depression and then let the particular disease class determine the treatment, or should we make the decision on treatment on the state of the patient once we have agreed that he falls into the general class of 'depression'? The first choice might be called treating the disease, and the second, treating the patient. According to the work of Carney and his colleagues (11), it is the second choice that yields the best results. This follows the classical advice of the medical teacher. Our present knowledge therefore suggests that the process of 'diagnosis' in the sense of allocation to a disease class should proceed sufficiently far so that a decision on treatment can be calculated on the patient's state. The problem remains of how this allocation of a patient to a disease class, 'diagnosis' in a restricted sense, is to be accomplished.

Diagnostic Inference

The process of inference is that whereby the probability of a hypothesis is altered in the light of evidence which is elicited. The hypothesis in this situation is that a certain disease is present and the method of inference which has been most commonly used is that based on the use of Bayes theorem (12). The probability we want is that of the disease given the evidence; that is, the set of symptoms, signs and laboratory findings, etc., each element of evidence being called an indicant. To calculate this probability, we need to know the initial probability of the disease and the probability of finding any indicant given that disease. These probabilities are connected as follows:

$$P(D_i|I_j) \propto P(D_i).P(I_j|D_i) \qquad \ldots 3$$

where D_i is the ith disease and I_j is the jth indicant. By the initial probability is meant the probability that the disease will be encountered in that particular area of clinical practice, an out-patient department for instance. The probability of any indicant, given a disease, is called a likelihood, and this requires a prospective study of a series of patients suffering from that disease. From such a sample, an estimate of the likelihood can be obtained. Formula 3 can be converted into an equation by making the right-hand side the numerator and putting as denominator the sum of all such expressions for all diseases.

$$P(D_i|I_j) = \frac{P(D_i).P(I_j|D_i)}{\Sigma_i P(D_i).P(I_j|D_i)} \qquad \ldots 4$$

This calculation is for a single indicant but the process is sequential and, as each fresh piece of evidence is elicited, the probability is recalculated for each disease in the set under consideration.

On paper the method appears straightforward and it has proved powerful and robust in practice. In certain areas it has proved about as good as a consultant specialising in that field (see, for example, References 13, 14, 15, 16, 17). This success is a little surprising. The assumption usually made by most workers who have used Bayesian inference is that the indicants they have elicited are statistically independent. By this is meant that, given the disease, the presence of one indicant does not alter the probability of finding another. Now to any experienced doctor this general assumption is manifestly false. It is in fact these sets of indicants which are statistically dependent *within one disease but not within another* that form the basis for the characteristic clinical patterns doctors learn to recognize. So it is somewhat surprising that the Bayesian method assuming independence is as good as it appears to be. It may be that much unnecessary evidence has been requested and that this excess compensates for the failure to use dependent probabilities. While dependent probabilities can be readily used in a Bayesian system a difficulty lies in their estimation from what are small samples (18). Where a comparison has been made between different methods of diagnostic inference, the Bayesian method appears to be as powerful as any (19) and the sequential calculation of the set of probabilities of the diseases under consideration is computationally straightforward and fits in well with the usual practice of the doctor.

Prognostic Inference; Estimation

Given a particular patient, there is a set of treatments, and corresponding to each of them, a set of outcomes. Mathematically, the prognosis is the probability of a given outcome for a given treatment in a given patient and may be symbolized as:

$$P(O_i|T_j,\underset{\sim}{X})$$

where O_i is the ith outcome, T_j is the jth treatment, and $\underset{\sim}{X}$ represents the vector which describes the patient. It is preferable, but not always possible, to calculate the probability in terms of the individual patient and not in terms of the 'disease' from which he is suffering.

The process of acquiring evidence to alter the probability of the hypothesis, that the patient will fall into a certain outcome class, may be called prognostic inference. But whereas in diagnostic inference, evidence is necessarily elicited sequentially, the estimate of a prognosis can frequently be made on evidence which has already been collected for diagnosis.

Estimation.

1. If a statistician is asked to estimate the set of prognoses, that is, the set of probabilities in a given situation, he might suggest that an informative experiment be carried out. In such an experiment a sample of patients would be collected, the set of treatments would be allocated randomly and the outcome in each case noted. Given sufficient data, the statistician would then be able to make estimates of the prognoses. Though this is perhaps the ideal method, it is not always permissible, since doctors may have some prior information of the outcomes so that it would be unethical to carry out a rigorous statistical procedure. This

procedure may, however, be justified with a new drug and then goes under the name of a therapeutic clinical trial.

2. Where the doctors participating in a trial, from their prior information, refuse to withhold a treatment for a particular type of patient, this refusal appears to invalidate the trial completely but Lindley (20) has shown how much information is still obtainable from such a trial.

3. Where there is a choice of treatments, it may not always be practicable to carry out an informative experiment. For example, for the results of surgical operation, a long follow-up of several years may be necessary. If it is desirable to institute formal methods of calculating treatment, some other method of arriving more rapidly at the set of prognoses is needed. One method might be to use the subjective probabilities of a panel of experts who simply rely on their experience. It would then be possible, from these prognoses, to calculate those factors in the patient's record and the weights to be attached to them, which would best predict the outcomes which occurred. Such weights could then be used on a prospective sample. The method, in effect, extracts the expertise of the panel.

4. There will be occasions when only one treatment is employed, the best available treatment, and here no decision problem arises since there is no choice of treatment. But it may be desirable for purposes of medical research or on other grounds to know the probability of the outcome of an individual patient.

The statistical methods employed are various and include the use of a linear discriminant function. In this a retrospective sample is taken where the outcomes are already known and those factors are selected which are believed to be relevant to the outcome. For example, in the prognosis of myocardial infarction, the factors might include age, a previous history of infarction, the degree of shock, the presence of a conduction defect and so on. The two outcomes are survival and death (21). Each factor has to be measured in each patient and then appropriately weighted and, by their sum, a single score obtained. This is done on the retrospective sample of patients and we imagine the scores for the 'survival' group and for the 'death' group to be normally distributed, and that each has the same variance. The two distributions are shown in Fig. 12.3. If we want to separate them we can do so by moving them apart, that is, maximizing the difference between their means, or by reducing the variance, or by both methods. In other words we wish to maximize $(m_1 - m_2)/s^2$. The statistical method of linear discrimination chooses the weights that do this. These weights can then be applied to individuals in a fresh sample to predict their outcomes though it will be found that, with a different sample, the prediction is less accurate.

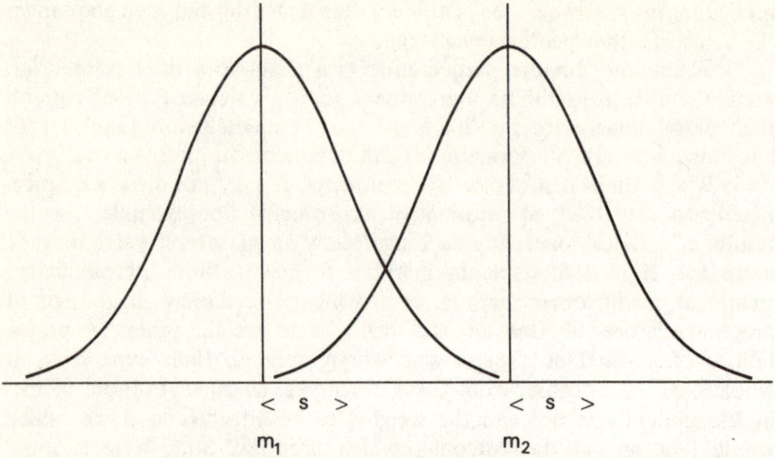

Figure 12.3. Distribution of scores for two groups: 'survival' group and 'death' group

Economic Relevance of These Ideas

The above outlines a scheme of formalized medicine using the techniques of probability and decision theory and the power of the computer, a scheme which has only become possible in the last 25 years. The computer has been used mainly as a calculating machine making mathematical methods possible which were previously quite impossible. Undoubtedly the most important, and at present the most difficult, part is the expression of the activities of clinical medicine in mathematical form and the computer plays an essential but secondary role. Much research in this field has fallen into the error that doctors know exactly how traditional medicine can and should be analysed and that all that is necessary to formalize it is to introduce the computer. This error has proved quite disastrous and in Britain has caused the waste of several million pounds (22).

The computer has usually been used as a calculating machine but could be used in its own right to do things which no purely calculating machine can do. An example is the use of a computer to play the game of checkers where it acquired a prodigious skill by playing thousands of games against itself, learning from its own mistakes. An application of this kind is theoretically possible in medicine. But, however the computer is used and whatever partnership is formed between man and the machine, the special skills of each should be used. Human beings are particularly skilled at very rapid pattern recognition, whether visual or auditory, and this skill is much used in medicine. Computers can store enormous amounts of data to which they have very rapid access, can calculate with great speed, do not fatigue and do not become confused, as do humans, by too much data.

The coming opportunities afforded by a formalized medicine are likely to force us to reconsider the traditional role of the doctor and indeed the whole organization of medical care. What has traditionally been done by the doctor has now to be questioned, even whether it really needs to be done by a doctor at all. In a formalized system of medicine which in effect uses a cost/benefit approach, the criteria that concern us are the accuracy of the data elicited from the patient; the power of the methods of inference and ultimately the accuracy of the decisions arrived at; the acceptability of the method to the patient; and the cost, in a National Health Service, to the community. While it is not possible to peer too far into the future it is already possible to foresee with some clarity changes in clinical medicine which could be realized within the next few years.

Computer-assisted Diagnosis. A good deal of work has been done in this field and has proved most useful in demonstrating how powerful are methods of inference, usually Bayesian, in making a diagnosis in the restricted sense. Its useful future is not clear unless the techniques of test reduction are adopted and the method extended to include decisions on management.

Computer Interrogation. Eliciting symptoms from a patient will be necessary for a very long while as symptoms are frequently the earliest manifestation of disease. These complaints of the patient have traditionally been elicited by the doctor by a process known as 'history taking'. Could this activity be assumed by the computer?

In 'history taking' the doctor obtains a number of facts about the patient's previous and present illness, but during all this questioning, the patient provides a stream of non-verbal information by his attitude, his gestures, his tone of voice, etc; but to questioning by the computer all this information is denied. It is therefore necessary to distinguish such questioning by using a different word, such as 'interrogation'. Where computer interrogation is confined to what may be called routine questioning in which non-verbal information is slight or unimportant, it appears that the computer is about as accurate as the doctor (23), and the method is as acceptable or possibly more acceptable to the patient (24). The usual method using a single mode of questioning could be improved by using both visual and auditory modes simultaneously and this is likely to result in better comprehension. But to confine the method to simple interrogation and a print-out of a list of symptoms is to fail completely to exploit the great potential of the method. There is no difficulty in principle in programing the computer to compute the set of probabilities of the diseases under consideration and these could be printed out at the end of interrogation. But it is possible to see even further. History taking is traditionally followed by physical examination of the patient and it is possible that in some situations this might be done by paramedical staff. The disease probabilities would then be recalculated. In theory it is now possible, and it may become possible in practice, to calculate the further tests which are advisable. If these calculations were done and the tests performed, the patient could see the doctor with much of the necessary evidence already elicited, together with a set of diagnostic probabilities and perhaps even suggestions on treatment. The ultimate decision on treatment has, of course, always to be made by a doctor.

Computer interrogation elicits evidence from the patient on which decisions may be made, some of which have been indicated. But there are others. When the diagnostic class is already known, for example, as in alcoholism, it may be possible to calculate the best treatment class using the opinions of a panel of experts to construct a decision tree, either probabilistic or deterministic. Multivariate statistical techniques exist for extracting and weighting the criteria which the experts are implicitly using but of which they may not be explicitly aware. While such a decision tree is not necessarily optimal, it would embody current expertise and would be generally available.

Test Reduction. The word 'test' usually refers to some laboratory examination, but it is used here in a more general sense to describe any method of eliciting information from a patient so that a question is a test as is a cardiac or radiological examination. There is considerable evidence that doctors use an unnecessary number of tests in their examination of a patient. This is not a criticism of the doctor since all human beings find it very difficult to assess evidence and estimate probabilities correctly. To know when a further test supplies fresh evidence rather than evidence which is already contained in the results of previous tests, is almost impossible. The assessment of evidence and the estimation of probabilities reached is very difficult for any human being even with special training. When, however, as in a formalized system of medicine, evidence can be measured, the effect on the set of probabilities of adding a further test to the set already used can be analysed. Where this has been done, very great reduction in the number of tests has been shown to be possible and the percentage reduction (though this measurement is not completely meaningful) ranges from 30 to 90 per cent. Since the sequence of tests traditionally done roughly follows their cost, a considerable saving should be possible, since the tests that can be omitted are frequently those that are done later in the sequence (25) – usually the more elaborate and therefore the more expensive ones.

Medical Records. A corollary of test reduction is the economy possible in recording medical information of an illness when the record is considered in the light of decision theory; that is, the information that may be needed to make decisions in some possible future illness. From unpublished work (26), it appears that a very condensed summary of the patient's illness can normally provide all the evidence necessary and that a very large reduction in the amount of information now recorded and stored is possible.

Self-medication. It is calculated that in Britain over 60 per cent of all symptoms are initially treated by the patient and this is done without skilled help (27). But it should be possible to develop decision trees devised by experts, to guide the layman in his self-treatment and to decide when he should consult a doctor. It is for experiment to measure the dangers and other costs of the method and benefits such as savings, and so determine what part it might usefully play in a Health Service (28).

Application of a Formalized Medicine to Developing Countries

The personal therapeutic system of medicine that we take for granted in the West is inapplicable to much of the world on account of its expense. A system of medicine is needed that does not depend so heavily on an expensively trained doctor. A possible alternative is by the use of decision trees in the hands of trained non-medical staff which concentrate on those conditions for which clear therapeutic gains are obtainable. Essex (29) has shown how effective such a method can be in Tanzania. Such decision trees have been constructed by an expert or group of experts using their insight and experience and are clearly most effective. They may, however, be suboptimal, and optimal decision trees could in principle be calculated. We do not yet know how useful this kind of approach is likely to be but the preliminary results are very encouraging.

References

1. Card, W.I. and Good, I.J. (1970). *Mathematical Biosciences,* **6**, 45.
2. Hull, J., Moore, P.G. and Thomas, H. (1973). *Journal of the Royal Statistical Society,* A, **136**, 226.
3. Card, W.I., Rusinkiewicz, M. and Phillips, C.I. (1976). *Decision Making and Medical Care.* Amsterdam, North-Holland Publishing.
4. Neumann, J. von and Morgenstern, O. (1953). *Theory of Games and Economic Behavior.* Princeton, University Press; Chichester, Wiley.
5. Weisbrod, B.A. (1961). *Journal of Political Economy,* **59**, 425.
6. Dawson, R.F.F. (1967). "Cost of Road Accidents in Great Britain" Road Research Laboratory, Ministry of Transport RLL Report, LR 79, Crowthorne.
7. Dawson, R.F.F. (1971). "Current Costs of Road Accidents in Great Britain" Road Research Laboratory, Department of the Environment RLL Report, LR396, Crowthorne.
8. Cohen of Birkenhead (1965-66). *Transactions of the Medical Society of London,* **82**, 181.
9. Cohen, H. (1943). *The Nature Method and Purpose of Diagnosis.* Cambridge, University Press.
10. Sneath, P.H.A. and Sokal, R.R. (1973). *Numerical Taxonomy: the Principles and Practice of Numerical Classification.* San Francisco, W.H. Freeman.

11. Carney, M.W.P., Roth, M. and Garside, R.F. (1965). *British Journal of Psychiatry,* **111**, 659.
12. Lindley, D. (1971). *Making Decisions.* New York and Chichester, Interscience.
13. Overall, J.E. and Williams, C.M. (1963). *Journal of the American Medical Association,* **183**, 307.
14. de Dombal, F.T., Leaper, D.J., Horrocks, J.C., Staniland, J.R. and McCann, A.P. (1974). *British Medical Journal,* **1**, 376.
15. de Dombal, F.T., Clamp, S.E., Leaper, D.J., Staniland, J.R. and Horrocks, J.C. (1975). *Gastroenterology,* **68**, 252.
16. Stern, R.B., Knill-Jones, R.P. and Williams, R. (1974). *Methods of Information in Medicine,* **13**, 79.
17. Stern, R.B., Knill-Jones, R.P. and Williams, R. (1975). *British Medical Journal,* **2**, 659.
18. Templeton, A.W., Jansen, C., Lehr, J.L. and Hufft, R. (1967). *Radiology,* **89**, 605.
19. Nordyke, R.A., Kulikowski, C.A. and Kulikowski, C.W. (1971). *Computers and Biomedical Research,* **4**, 374.
20. Lindley, D.V. (1975). *Journal of the Royal Statistical Society (C),* **24**, 218.
21. Hughes, W.L., Kalbfleisch, J.M., Brandt, E.N. and Costiloe, J.P. (1963). *Archives of Internal Medicine,* **111**, 338.
22. Committee on Public Accounts (1976). *Sixth Report,* paras. 105-118. London, HMSO.
23. Card, W.I., Nicholson, M., Crean, G.P., Watkinson, G., Evans, C.R., Wilson, J. and Russell, D. (1974). *International Journal of Bio-Medical Computing,* **5**, 175.
24. Lucas, R.W., Card, W.I., Knill-Jones, R.P., Watkinson, G. and Crean, G.P. (1976). *British Medical Journal,* **2**, 623.
25. Computer Committee Report. *Test Reduction.* London, Royal College of Physicians. (In preparation).
26. Card, W.I., Sircus, W. and Smith, A.N. (In preparation).
27. OHE (1968). "Without Prescription; a Study of the Role of Self-medication" Number 27. London, Office of Health Economics.
28. Backett, E.M. and England, R. (1975). *Lancet,* **ii**, 1137.
29. Essex, B.J. (1975). *British Medical Journal,* **3**, 34.

13

Decision Making and Cost-benefit Analysis in Medicine

Sir Michael Woodruff

So many people are involved in decision making in medicine, and their decisions interact in such a complex way, that it would be a formidable task to attempt a detailed analysis and the dividends might well be meagre in comparison with the effort involved. It may nevertheless be useful to define some of the main areas in which decisions are made, and examine in broad outline the ways in which decisions in one area may influence the options available in others.

Let us begin by considering an individual's decision to consult a doctor; to become, in short, a patient. This choice of starting point is a matter of convenience rather than logical necessity, for it presupposes that there are doctors to consult, and the truth of this supposition depends on prior decision by other individuals and by health and education authorities of various kinds. Moreover, a person's illness or injury may be such that a decision to seek medical advice on his behalf will have been taken by others.

A person who seeks medical advice, as distinct from a routine examination for life insurance or similar purposes, does so because he has experienced symptoms which have, or which he fears may have, unpleasant consequences in the form of pain, incapacity or shortened life expectancy; and he seeks treatment, or some form of prognosis, or both. The qualification in respect of prognosis is important because many patients would not welcome an immediate completely frank statement if the prognosis were poor; it would, on the other hand, be pointless to seek reassurance if one knew in advance that this would always be given however grave the true prognosis might be.

Having decided to seek medical advice the patient has next to decide how urgently he should do this and to whom he should go.

Many factors influence these decisions, including the patient's personal assessment of the significance of his symptoms, which may be far wide of the mark; his fear of hearing bad news when, rightly or wrongly, this is what he expects; and, sometimes, his reluctance to bother his doctor, when, again rightly or wrongly, he suspects that his symptoms are not of serious import.

How can people be helped to decide wisely? Education of the public in matters medical can be useful, especially by alerting people to potentially dangerous symptoms, as is illustrated, for example, by the reduction in the death rate from malignant melanoma in Queensland following publicity concerning the possible danger of black spots. In this as in other contexts, however, a little learning can be dangerous, and people should be encouraged to seek advice promptly about unusual symptoms, and not rely on their own judgement as to whether or not these are important. A corollary of this proposition is that doctors should adopt a sympathetic attitude to sincere patients even when their fears prove groundless or even appear absurd, like those of the young man who woke me up when I was a Casualty Officer because he felt something moving in his chest, and having been told that this was his heart and would continue to beat throughout his life, woke me up again a week later in a state of panic because he was now afraid that his heart had stopped beating.

The patient's choice of where to go for advice often appears to be made almost at random, and it is not easy to remedy this situation. It is usually wise, despite occasional much publicized instances pointing to the contrary, to avoid unregistered quacks, but how should a patient choose between one general practitioner and another? This may be quite easy for a doctor who becomes a patient himself, if he has lived long enough in a place to have had an opportunity of assessing the professional competence of his colleagues, but it is a very different matter for the layman. There is no obvious solution to the problem, but it merits more serious study by both doctors and laymen than it has yet received.

Similar considerations arise when relatives, friends or bystanders have to seek advice on behalf of someone else, except that there is then unlikely to be much doubt whether or not advice is needed.

When a general practitioner is consulted he has to decide what to tell the patient about his condition and what advice to give concerning treatment. Should he offer to treat the patient himself, and, if so, what should he prescribe; alternatively, should he refer the patient to a specialist colleague, and, if so, to whom? Sometimes the practitioner's choice of consultant seems, like the patient's choice of practitioner, to be made almost at random, but for this there is clearly no excuse. Similar decisions about what to tell the patient, and what treatment to advise, have to be made by consultants, but with the difference that it is in general less easy for the consultant to pass the responsibility on to someone else.

To make wise decisions a doctor, whether general practitioner or consultant, needs knowledge and experience, but these qualifications are not enough. He needs also to be deeply concerned about his patient but at the same time to maintain a measure of detachment – *aequanimitas* as Osler called it – and he must be prepared to make decisions on the basis of the evidence obtainable in a period of time commensurate with the urgency of the condition, even when this evidence is insufficient to be conclusive. The decision, for example, whether or not to open a child's abdomen in the middle of the night, or whether to attempt a radical operation in a patient with cancer or to settle for a palliative procedure, may have very important consequences but may have to be taken on evidence which would be regarded as inadequate by a scientist or even a lawyer.

Decisions about what to tell patients are important in relation to treatment because, while it is open to any patient who is conscious, of sound mind and old enough to decide important questions on his own account, to accept or reject his doctor's advice, the extent to which a patient can contribute to wise decision making depends on how much he knows about his condition and about the probable outcome of various possible courses of action including the one recommended by his doctor. It is, in my view, always wrong to lie to a patient, but it is surely right to edit the truth and tell him no more than he is ready, or needs, to know. And if a patient refrains from asking direct questions it may be proper to withhold bad news indefinitely provided that this does not affect decisions about treatment. When, however, treatment which the doctor regards as important is refused, it is essential to make sure that the patient is aware of why this treatment was advised, and what is likely to happen if it is, or is not, accepted. If a patient with an apparently operable cancer in the lower rectum is told that he has 'a small ulcer' and refuses on this account to submit to abdominoperineal resection, it is not the patient who is behaving irrationally but the doctor; the patient should be told the true nature of his condition and the advantages of prompt surgical treatment.

With unconscious patients the doctor may have to decide whether to start artificial respiration, and, if this is started but the patient is found subsequently to have irreversible brain damage which will prevent him from ever regaining consciousness or breathing spontaneously, when to switch off the respirator. The next of kin and other close relatives should, as far as possible, be kept informed of the situation, but the decision to put a patient on a respirator has to be taken urgently with little time for consultation, and the decision to switch off must, in the last resort, be taken by the doctor in charge after consultation with appropriate colleagues.

While the primary responsibility of a general practitioner or consultant is to individual patients, this is not the whole story. I have discussed the matter at length elsewhere (1); suffice it to say, therefore, that the categories of people the doctor may have to consider include the patient's relatives, other people directly at risk as the result of the patient's illness or incapacity, coroners and procurators fiscal, and people who at some future time may develop the same kind of disease as the patient. Moreover, modern treatment is often a matter of teamwork, so that medical colleagues, nurses, laboratory and social workers, and others may participate to a greater or lesser extent in decisions about patient management.

Finally, there is an area of decision making of great importance which can be categorized as administrative. Decisions in this area are not, or should not be, concerned with the management of particular patients by methods which are in general use; they are concerned with the priorities to be observed in making new resources available, in deploying doctors and other medical workers in the community, and, to some extent at least, in research. It is important that such decisions should be based on reliable evidence and on sound advice from clinicians and medical scientists; that they should be expressed in unambiguous terms; and that responsibility for their consequences should be accepted, and be seen to be accepted, by those making the decisions. It is deplorable that individual clinicians should sometimes be thought by their patients to be responsible for deficiencies in standards of care which are the direct consequence of administrative decisions in which the clinicians concerned have played no part, or which they may even have opposed.

It is obviously desirable that available resources should be used to the best advantage, and it is therefore right that, in principle, administrative decisions should take account of estimates of cost effectiveness; in practice, however, this is not easy to achieve. Analysis of costs, though a demanding task, does not pose any new problems unique to medical, as distinct from other forms of, administration; but how should effectiveness be measured?

The first difficulty is to define the possible beneficiaries. It seems clear that, if treatment can properly be described as successful, the beneficiaries include the patient himself; but if we agree with Donne that 'any man's death diminishes me' then we must think in wider terms. It would, however, be absurd to suppose that the world was equally afflicted by the deaths of, let us say, Mozart and Hitler, or that a family is afflicted to the same extent by the chronic illness of a young mother or the death of a mongol child or an aged grandparent. To complicate matters further the struggle of an individual in the face of adversity may provide inspiration for others. In one way the world would have been poorer if medical science had advanced to such a point that Helen Keller's affliction had been cured in early life; on the other hand, children similarly afflicted, but lacking her ability to triumph in the face of disaster, and, many would say, Helen Keller herself, would have benefited from such treatment. But how can one even begin to quantify such imponderables?

One way of avoiding getting lost in this maze is to refuse to enter it; in other words, to consider only benefit to the individual patient. This is in fact what, to a close degree of approximation, most practising doctors do. In my view this is a sound tradition and I have always felt uneasy about the suggestion, at one time seriously advanced in relation to the treatment of patients with irreversible renal failure when facilities for haemodialysis and renal transplantation were even less adequate in relation to the demand than they are today, that patients should be selected on the basis of their supposed value to the community. The alternative which I have adopted, and which I would defend on the ground that it results in fewer anomalies than any other procedure, is to select patients primarily on the basis of whether they are likely to benefit significantly from the treatment, and then proceed on the basis of first come first served.

Even when we consider only the direct benefit of treatment to individual patients, however, quantification is not easy. This is true even in the hypothetical model of the population of indistinguishable individuals, each suffering from the same disease, because one must consider not only length of survival but also the quality of life enjoyed by each patient; with a heterogeneous population of real patients, suffering from a great variety of disorders, the problem of quantifying benefit becomes incomparably more difficult.

A course of action which is right for practising doctors is not necessarily right for administrators or community physicians, who must, perforce, look beyond the individual patient. They cannot, therefore, keep out of the maze but, having entered, they would be wise to explore it a little bit at a time.

The first step, after considering individual patients, might well be to consider all these currently healthy people who benefit from the assurance that appropriate treatment will be available for them should they ever become ill. It is not only the person whose house actually catches fire who benefits from the existence of the fire brigade.

In medicine, the extent to which the community will benefit in this way may be increased both by making more effective use of current knowledge and by extending the frontier of knowledge through research. Once again costing, in principle, raises no special problem, but assessment of benefit is very difficult; and prediction of the benefit likely to accrue from a particular research project is more difficult still. It is important to notice, however, that the 'fire brigade' type of benefit is not as closely related to the incidence of particular diseases as is the benefit experienced by patients receiving treatment. Only the comparatively small number of patients who actually receive a kidney transplant, or undergo open heart surgery, or are treated in a coronary care unit, can be said to benefit from such treatment, but every member of a community in which these forms of treatment are generally available benefits from the assurance of their availability.

It follows from what has been said that it would be naive to suppose that we shall ever develop a rigorous calculus of cost-benefit analysis in relation to medicine. It would nevertheless be disastrous to abandon the attempt to achieve this, for one of the mainsprings of human progress – perhaps indeed the only one – is man's struggle to reach unattainable goals.

Reference

1. Woodruff, M.F.A. (1970). *The One And The Many*. London, Royal Society of Medicine.
Reprinted in *On Science and Surgery*. (1976). Edinburgh, University Press.

Part Three
Drugs

14

Prescribing

O.L. Wade

The National Health Service Act 1946 provides for the supply of 'proper and sufficient drugs and medicines' and it is a doctor's duty by regulations made under that Act to prescribe whatever drugs are required for the proper treatment of his patient. The principle that there should be no restriction of the prescribing by a doctor of any drug which is in his opinion necessary for the treatment of his patients was accepted by Parliament and has since been jealously guarded by the medical profession, but it is accepted that the doctor should exercise reasonable care in avoiding waste of public funds.

There has, however, been deep concern about the costs of the pharmaceutical services from the inception of the National Health Service. Five governmental enquiries on prescribing costs have been conducted in the last 25 years (1, 2, 3, 4, 5) and numerous authors and editors have explored the subject with varying degrees of objectivity and emotion.

This chapter is concerned with the cost of prescribing and the prices of ethical drugs. An 'ethical preparation', an inappropriate phrase of American provenance, is one that is normally obtained by patients only with a doctor's prescription and is not advertised directly to the public.

In the National Health Service drugs are prescribed by doctors working in hospitals and in general practice. Wade and Elmes have shown that in Northern Ireland the cost of drugs used in the hospital service was only 4 or 5 per cent of the total drug bill. The remaining 95 or 96 per cent of the cost of the pharmaceutical services was for the prescribing by family doctors in general practice. The situation is likely to be similar in England and Wales and in Scotland.

*The Cost of the NHS Pharmaceutical Services**

In the first year for which figures are available, 1949/50, the cost of the pharmaceutical services in England and Wales was £31 million, and by 1957/58 this had doubled to £62 million. This was 8 per cent of the cost of the whole service in 1949/50 and 10 per cent in 1957/58. In 1974 (Table 14.1) the expenditure on the pharmaceutical services for England,

Table 14.1

Pharmaceutical services, 1974.	
Total NHS expenditure	£4300 million (estimated)
Pharmaceutical services	£ 359 million
Prescriptions issued	£ 294 million
Average cost per prescription	99p
Average number of prescriptions per head of population	6.0
Pharmaceutical industry – value of sales, 1975	
To NHS	£ 344 million
To exports	£ 373 million (£104 million in first 3 months 1976)
To household remedies	£ 120 million
Value of imported drugs	£ 97 million
Estimate of research and development costs of pharmaceutical industry	£ 70 million

From ABPI Annual Report 1975/76 and ABPI News Bulletin May 1976.

Wales and Scotland was £359 million. This was 8.5 per cent of the total cost of the National Health Service. However, the cost of drugs has increased relative to other expenses since that time and the pharmaceutical services in 1975 and 1976 were again about 10 per cent of the total NHS expenditure (provisional figures and estimates) as has been the case for most of the last 20 years.

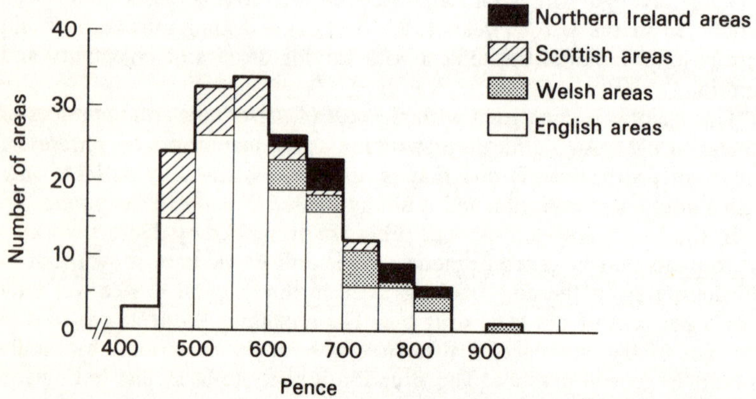

Figure 14.1 Prescribing costs in general practice. Distribution of areas by average total cost per person – United Kingdom, 1974. (From Government of Northern Ireland (5).)

It is, however, known that the expenditure on drugs varies greatly in different parts of the United Kingdom. In 1964* the average cost for pharmaceutical services varied from 400-449 (old) pence per person in three areas of England to 900-950 (old) pence per person in one area of Scotland (Fig. 14.1). The mean figures for England, Wales, Scotland and Northern Ireland showed considerable differences (Table 14.2). In general, the cost of prescribing was highest in areas that were economically backward and where unemployment was highest. Unfortunately, it was not

Table 14.2
Average costs per prescription and per person, 1964

	England	*Wales*	*Scotland*	*Northern Ireland*
Average cost per prescription (old pence)				
Net ingredient cost	81.6	90.3	83.5	93.8
Distribution costs	38.7	40.0	41.4	44.9
Total cost	120.3	130.3	124.9	138.7
Average number of prescriptions per person	4.58	5.62	4.28	5.19
Average cost per person (old pence)				
Ingredient cost	373.5	507.5	357.3	486.9
Distribution cost	177.4	225.1	177.5	232.9
Total cost	550.9	732.6	534.8	719.8

From Government of Northern Ireland (5).

possible to relate the costs of prescribing to the age and sex structure of the population, the morbidity rates or the mortality rates in the different areas (5).

Differences in the Prescribing of Drugs

There have been very few published studies of the prescribing of drugs by doctors. Those which have been undertaken show that marked changes of the pattern of prescribing may take place over relatively short periods of time. Figures 14.2 and 14.3 show the changes in the prescribing of hypnotics and bronchodilators by doctors in general practice in Northern Ireland. Even more interesting is that the patterns of prescribing by doctors

*Throughout this chapter I have been handicapped by the problem of obtaining suitable data on which to base comparisons. I have often had to use data which was older than I wished, for there is a great time lag in the publication of many statistics and recent data may not be available in suitable form.

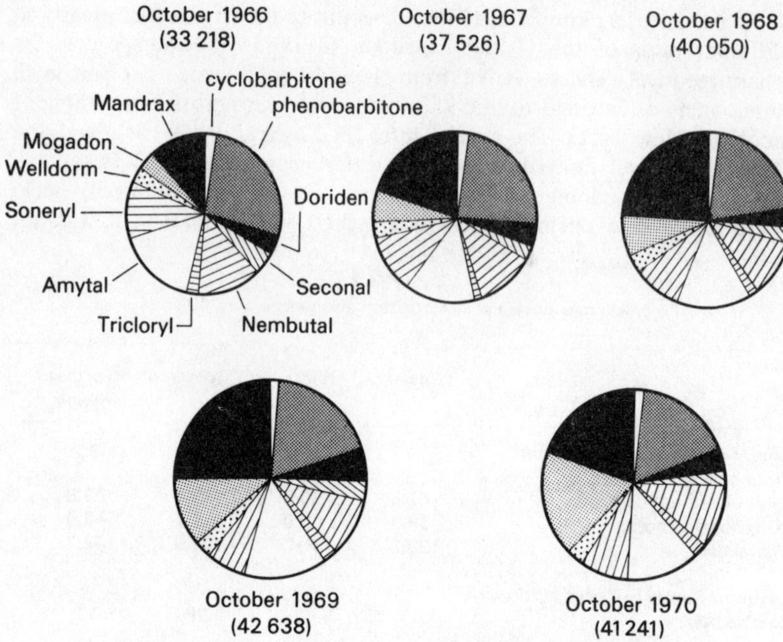

Figure 14.2. Prescribing of hypnotic drugs in Northern Ireland, 1966-1970.

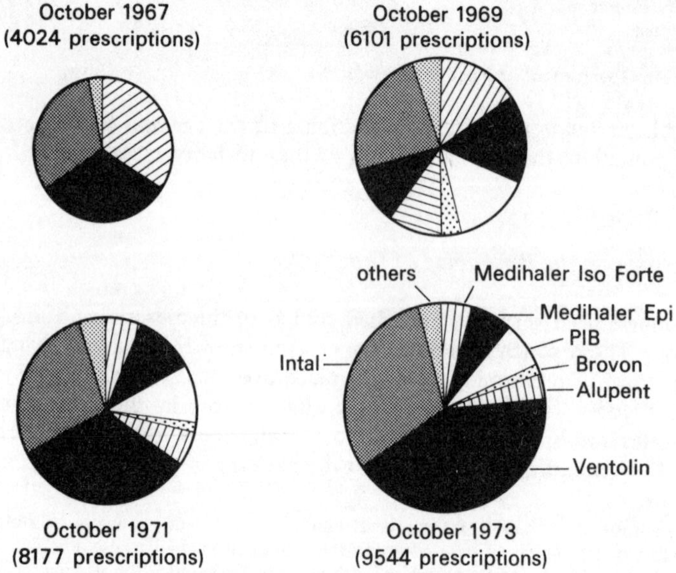

Figure 14.3. Prescribing of bronchodilators in Northern Ireland, 1967-1973.

may vary geographically. Wade (6) found that although the prescribing of insulin was remarkably constant per 1,000 patients on doctors' lists per unit of time, there were great differences in different parts of Northern Ireland in the prescribing of oral hypoglycaemic drugs (Fig. 14.4), thyroid

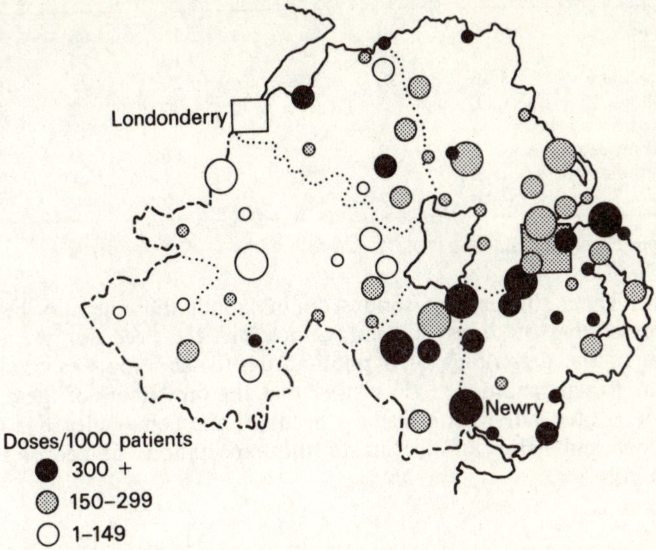

Figure 14.4. Prescribing of oral hypoglycaemic drugs in Northern Ireland, 1966. The squares represent Belfast and Londonderry. The circles represent the centres of population, the size of the circle being proportional to the population.

and antithyroid drugs and antihypertensive drugs. More recently it has been shown (7, 8) that there are very great differences in the prescribing of hypnotics in different areas of the Province. In the whole Province, on average, 42 doses of hypnotic drugs were prescribed each day for every 1,000 patients on doctors' lists, but in the residential areas of Belfast and adjoining County Down the average was 76.6 doses/1,000 patients/day, and in Fermanagh, Londonderry City and Londonderry County the average was 23.5-24.7 doses/1,000 persons/day. Studies in Norway and Sweden have confirmed that similar differences of prescribing occur from area to area (9).

Differences between countries may be even more marked than differences within a country. One of the first international studies of the differences in the use of drugs between countries was carried out by Engels and Siderius (10), who examined the sales of antibiotics in six European countries (Table 14.3). Studies by a WHO Working Party on Drug Consumption have since shown that there are marked differences in the prescribing of oral anticoagulants, vitamin B_{12}, antihypertensive drugs and oral hypoglycaemic drugs (9) in Norway, Sweden and Northern

Table 14.3
Sales of antibiotics in Europe, 1966-1967
(percentage of total sales within each country)

	France	UK	West Germany	Belgium	Sweden	Holland
Penicillin	20	35	45	11	55	30
Ampicillin	1	15	5	13	15	30
Tetracyclines	40	35	20	20	25	30
Macrolides	8	5	1	30	2	2
Combined macrolides and tetracyclines	8	2	1	15	0	1
Chloramphenicol	5	1	25	1	1	1
Others	18	7	3	10	2	6

From Engels and Siderius (10).

Ireland. These studies raise serious doubts about the congruity between the prescribing of drugs in communities and the need for them. The studies of the prescribing of hypnotic drugs (8) and, more especially, of vitamin B_{12} preparations (11) suggest that the prescribing of these drugs may be related not to the medical needs of the community but to the traditions and habits of doctors or the expectations of people in the community.

The Price of Drugs

There has been for many years criticism of the price of drugs and the profits of the pharmaceutical industry. In the USA public confidence in the drug industry was profoundly shaken by the Kefauver hearings (12) which showed that some firms were unscrupulous in the marketing of drugs and charged prices related to 'what the market would bear' rather than to the costs of production. Companies were accused of making too much profit, using misleading advertisements, spending too much on advertising, using trademarks to keep up prices, conducting useless research, putting improper pressures on governmental agencies, selling ineffective or even dangerous products, failing to carry out appropriate tests, risking patients in clinical trials, exploiting research employees and over-compensating executives. Similar but less excessive criticism has been made in the UK and Europe. It has been rebutted with vigour by the drug industry which points to its record of innovation, the valuable contributions the industry makes to modern medicine and the enormous costs of research and development. It is estimated that the average expenditure on research and development for a completely new drug has risen from $1.4 million in the early 1950s to over $40 million in the 1970s (13). Moreover, the industry faces risks that are unusual compared with other industries, for a product on which a great deal has been spent may be made obsolescent very rapidly by some new discovery. The most quoted example of this is the replacement of the pneumococcal antisera almost as soon as they had been first produced in the late 1930s, by the sulphonamides. In the UK the pharmaceutical industry makes a major contribution to the national balance of payments. Products worth £221 million were exported in 1973; pharmaceutical imports were £66.9 million (Overseas Trade Statistics). The industry has defended the use of trade names vigorously because of their importance in the export trade.

One of the reasons that anxiety persists about the profits of the pharmaceutical industry is that there are serious doubts of how competitive drug prices are because in this industry there are firms which hold an almost exclusive trade of certain types of drugs, such as penicillins, corticosteroids and benzodiazepines. The recent decision by the Department of Health and Social Security to withhold payments to the Swiss based firm Hoffman-La-Roche, a decision upheld in a Court of Appeal, has not helped to assuage these doubts. There has been concern, too, about the policies that companies have about the development of new drugs. Some companies appear to be concerned more with the ultimate marketability of a new drug than the community's need for it. A new oral analgesic or minor tranquillizer will be pursued with keenness because the sales team believes, probably correctly, that such a new drug can be sold. It may be commercially difficult to market a drug that is of great importance to only a handful of people who suffer from a rare illness such as Wilson's disease. Dr Fattorusso (14), Director of Prophylactic Diagnostic and Therapeutic Substances in the World Health Organization, has recently complained that the pharmaceutical industries of the world in general take a negative attitude towards the development of tropical medicines because the financial returns from developing countries are low. There are, however, some firms in the UK which have made major contributions in this field.

The arguments about whether current drug prices are fair or excessive will continue, especially in a country which has a state health service which is the dominant purchaser of the output of ethical drugs. The economist has difficulty in assessing the situation, for the normal constraints of demand and supply in an open market do not apply. Ethical drugs are produced by industry, advertised to the medical profession, prescribed by doctors, consumed by patients and paid for mainly by the taxpayer. The state faces an array of parties interested in increasing the value and volume of drugs that are prescribed. The practitioner on behalf of his patient, and sometimes at the demand of his patient, is ready to prescribe medicines that he thinks are or may be efficacious and is himself insulated from any consideration of cost. The patient, also insulated from cost, is naturally anxious to get the most efficacious medicine and is likely to imagine that the newest and most expensive drugs are the ones he needs. The manufacturers or suppliers of medicines are anxious to sell as much as possible of their wares at as high a price as is possible. Price is not functioning to balance supply and demand, for high prices do not necessarily lead to a reduction in the manufacturer's monetary return. The distributors and dispensers of medicines, the pharmacists, also stand to benefit financially if the value and volume of their turn-over increases.

Advertising

There is nothing inherently evil about drug advertising. If a new and useful drug is marketed and is not promptly and properly prescribed for those patients who will benefit, then it is underused and the public may suffer.

The trouble with most sales promotion, however, is that it aims to persuade doctors to use particular preparations and, although seldom dishonest, it is often unduly optimistic. To the extent that it succeeds in persuading doctors to prescribe a new preparation which gives no benefit beyond those already available, or to prescribe it for patients who do not need it at all, then it encourages overuse of the drug, the public is ill served and the state defrauded.

There are three reasons why excessively optimistic advertising of drugs flourishes.

1. Most doctors are not experts in assessing the claims made by companies about their drugs; indeed the assessment of the effectiveness and value of a drug is a complex business which demands exceptional expertise. It is therefore relatively easy for a pharmaceutical salesman to persuade many doctors to prescribe the drugs he wishes to sell.
2. Useful and unbiased information about drugs, especially new drugs, is not available in a sufficiently accessible form.
3. Few of the leaders of the pharmaceutical industry, many of them dedicated, hardworking and fairminded, are doctors. They are men who devote their lives to producing drugs and are, understandably, strongly convinced of the benefits of drug therapy in disease. This conviction carries over to their sales force.

The company representatives who visit doctors are the most powerful advertising tool the drug industry has. More is spent on them than on any other form of advertising (Table 14.4). Even if a representative does not impress a doctor about an individual drug, he and his colleagues imperceptibly and possible unconscioully create an image of the effectiveness of drug therapy which is better than it should be. The expenditure on advertising in the UK far exceeds the present expenditure on postgraduate education of doctors. Abel-Smith (15) estimates that, for the cost of sales promotion, it would be possible for each general practitioner to have a teacher of medicine or therapeutics spend a month in his practice each year working with him and giving advice.

Although pharmaceutical companies foster the illusion that doctors are deeply concerned that their patients should receive specified brand

Table 14.4
Expenditure on advertising and sales promotion to doctors, 1961

Manufacturers' sales	£67 million	
		Percentage of sales
Mail advertising*	£1.85 million	2.8
Samples	£0.83 million	1.25
Journal advertising	£0.95 million	1.42
Estimated costs of representatives †	£2.90 million	4.34
	£6.57 million	9.78

Data from paper to Public Accounts Committee, House of Commons, 1962.
* Cost of advertising in journals for other professions – pharmacists, dentists, etc.: £0.13 million

† Total cost was £4.60 million but some of the work of representatives is promotion to chemists, inspecting stocks, etc.

products, enquiries suggest that doctors would usually be just as ready to use generic names if they were short, snappy and easy to remember. If a suitable, easily remembered code were put against each preparation in the British National Formulary there is no doubt that many doctors would use this when writing their prescription instead of using trade names.

Would Patients Suffer if Doctors Economized in their Prescribing?

Most observers would agree that in the UK at present considerable economy in prescribing is possible without patients suffering – indeed they would benefit. There are three areas where saving might be achieved, either by not prescribing at all or by prescribing simpler and less expensive drugs. These are where:

1. Valuable but expensive drugs such as antibiotics, corticosteroid ointments, antihypertensive drugs and psychotropic drugs are prescribed for illnesses which they are unlikely to help, or are prescribed in such a way that they are of little or no value.

2. Expensive proprietary preparations which have no proven virtue over simpler medicines, such as elegant cough mixtures or tonics, or which are of doubtful therapeutic value, such as the vasodilators promoted for the use of patients with strokes, are prescribed because they are aggressively advertised. Some of the proprietary compound preparations such as those containing barbiturates with amphetamines, analgesics or bronchodilators are not only expensive but are frankly undesirable.

3. Medicine-taking is fulfilling non-pharmacological functions. Medicines may be needed by a patient to justify the sick role he has adopted to himself or those around him. They may be needed so that a patient feels he or his doctor is doing something positive to make him better. Simple

and inexpensive medicines would fulfil the purpose as effectively as expensive medicines.

A lot of minor illness is self-limiting. If a medicine has been prescribed for a cold or a headache, when recovery takes place it may be ascribed by the patient and sometimes by the doctor to the medication and, when a similar illness recurs subsequently, medication is again demanded: in such a situation simple and inexpensive preparations will be as effective as expensive remedies if prescribed with appropriate confidence. It is, of course, not easy to estimate the prevalence of such situations: it probably varies from practice to practice and from doctor to doctor. There is considerable lack of unanimity amongst doctors about the proportion of patients who consult them who do not need to consult a doctor and could reasonably treat themselves with household remedies (16). Nevertheless there is wide agreement that the cost of prescribing could be cut substantially by most doctors if they were minded so to do.

The Attitude of the Doctor to Drug Costs

In those situations in which a doctor has to purchase drugs in order to dispense them himself, as is the case for a few doctors in the NHS, or in which his patients, who are not affluent, will have to pay for the drugs themselves, as was only too frequently the situation for elderly patients in the USA before the 'Medicare' scheme was introduced, doctors know the cost of drugs, are aware of the need for economy, and can and do prescribe economically. For most doctors in the NHS there is, however, little incentive to know the cost of the drugs they prescribe, and although there are many exceptions, most doctors give remarkably little thought to economy in their prescribing. Dunnell and Cartwright (16) sent a questionnaire to 581 doctors in the UK. Of the 326 who replied to the questionnaire, more than half of them thought they would write fewer prescriptions if they spent more time with their patients; one doctor said 'What people really want is to be listened to. Prescribing is rarely needed.' Elmes and his colleagues (8), however, found some evidence that doctors who had small lists tended to be the heaviest prescribers. It may be that even though a doctor decides the patient does not need a prescription, he finds it difficult not to give one, and if he spends longer with his patients he may learn of more symptoms and be under even greater pressure to prescribe than if his consultation is short.

How Could Economy of Prescribing be Achieved in the NHS?

There are at least nine methods which either have been used or might be used, alone or in combination, to achieve economies in prescribing.

1. *Influencing the Prescriber.* It is claimed that if medical students were taught more about the cost of drugs and the need for economy and if measures were sought to acquaint general practitioners and hospital consultants with a simple and striking form of the efficacy and relative costs of drugs, the prescribing costs of the NHS would be substantially reduced. Those who have had experience of undergraduate and graduate teaching, however, would not expect such efforts to be more than marginally effective. In education it is not what is taught that is important, it is what is learnt. Experience has shown that many doctors will learn readily enough about what they think is important to them, about drugs, the use of drugs, the mechanism of action of drugs or adverse reactions to drugs, but they cannot be expected to take a major interest in drug costs from which they are so insulated. The DHSS has for many years bombarded doctors with information about the cost of drugs, advised on equivalents or near equivalents to proprietary medicines, urged a preference of non-proprietary to proprietary medicines, exhorted the use of generic names instead of the more easily memorized trade names and arranged lectures to stiffen the resistance of doctors to the claims of advertisements and the persuasion of salesmen: but all to little effect. Indeed, it would be interesting to discover whether the DHSS can justify the costs of its campaigns by showing that they had led to substantial savings. The information about drug costs that they circulate seems unlikely to make much impact on doctors who are being simultaneously subjected to the deluge of advertisements from drug companies which pours through their letterbox, and the visits of persuasive salesmen.

2. *Disciplining the Prescriber.* Since 1950 the Pricing Bureau has at regular intervals analysed the prescribing costs of every doctor, who is informed of his costs in relation to the average of doctors in his area. Those whose prescribing costs are unduly high, usually more than twice the average of other doctors in the area, are visited by Regional Medical Officers. After such a visit doctors usually reduce the cost of their prescribing but if they persist they may be called to appear before a Local Medical Committee to justify their prescribing. The Local Medical Committee may advise that monies be withheld from a doctor's remuneration. This is a clumsy machinery and is seldom used except where there has been a gross or stupid abuse. The costs of carrying out the analyses and of visiting the doctors may not be justified by any reduction in the prescribing costs that result, for the system causes resentment and ill-feeling among some doctors and may be counter-productive in terms of their willingness to co-operate with the DHSS. There is a story about one doctor who was visited by a Regional Medical Officer. He subsequently wrote to the 3 per cent of patients on his lists for whom his prescribing had been most expensive, requesting them to transfer to other practices. He not only cut down his prescribing costs dramatically but he reduced his work-load by 25 per cent.

3. *Prescription Charges.* In 1952 a prescription charge was imposed. Initially it was 1 shilling per prescription form but in 1958 it was increased to a 1 shilling per item. The imposition of prescription charges was initially opposed vigorously by the British Medical Association, but when in 1963 there was a proposal that they should be abolished there was a *volte face;* anxiety that nothing should interfere with the supply of drugs that a patient needed had been replaced by anxiety that withdrawal of the charges would increase the number of unnecessary visits made to doctors for minor needs.

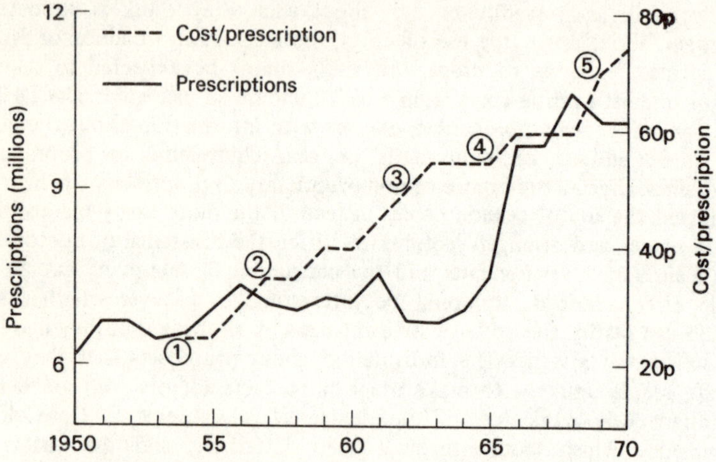

Figure 14.5. Prescriptions and the cost per prescription in Northern Ireland, 1950-1970. (1) 1s 0d per form (2) 1s 0d per item (3) 2s 0d per item (4) all charges abolished (5) 2s 6d per item

The graph (Fig. 14.5) shows that in Northern Ireland neither the imposition, the removal of prescription charges, their reimposition nor changes in the charges, seemed to make much difference to the rate of increase in the costs of prescribing over a period of 20 years. Indeed, on reflection, a fixed prescription charge dependent on the number of items prescribed would not be expected to have very much effect on the major cause of the increased drug bill which is the increased cost of each item. If the prescription charges were varied according to the cost of the drug, they might make some impact on the cost of prescribing but it would very fairly invite an accusation of charging the sick and would be politically unacceptable.

4. *Regulation of Drug Prices.* In 1957 the Ministry of Health entered into an agreement with the Association of the British Pharmaceutical Industry for a scheme of price regulation. The main features of the scheme were:

1. If a preparation had substantial exports the home price should be no more than the export price.

2. If a preparation, not substantially exported, had an exact standard equivalent its price should be no higher than the equivalent.

3. For other preparations the maximum price should be calculated by a specially constructed trade price formula.

New preparations were excluded from this scheme for four years if they were the results of research and for two if they were not.

By 1959 prices had been agreed for some 88 per cent by value of all preparations falling within the scope of the scheme.

This scheme, with modifications, has continued since. It is difficult to assess its efficacy but it would appear to have been very successful if the prices of drugs in the UK are compared with prices in other countries (Table 14.5). It works because both parties concerned wish the scheme

Table 14.5
Per capita expenditure on pharmaceuticals supplied through pharmacists (decimal pound sterling)

	1964	*1969*	*Increase*
Belgium	na	7.56	
Finland	na	4.60	
France	4.84	9.60	98%
Germany (West)	3.00	6.60	120%
Italy	2.54	6.25	146%
Japan	na	8.50	
Spain	2.12	4.43	109%
Turkey	na	0.99	
UK	2.20	3.38	54%

It is difficult to compare drug prices because exchange rates are a poor and uncertain reflection of purchasing power. Although in 1969 the UK apparently had the lowest per capita expenditure apart from Turkey, of more reliability and significance is that between 1964 and 1969 expenditure in the UK rose only 54% compared with 98-146% in other countries for which data is available. USA expenditure is not included but is dramatically higher than in Europe, because of the much higher wage rates in that country. (NEDO, 1972, International Price Comparison, National Economic Development Office.) (Reproduced by permission of the Controller of HMSO.)

to work. The State cannot demand prices so low that it exposes itself to the accusation that it has driven drugs off the market or has made the discovery of new drugs more difficult: the pharmaceutical industry cannot be indifferent to allegations that it is profiteering at the expense of the sick.

5. *Restrictions on Advertising.* Many believe that the excessive and insistent claims made in drug advertisements encourage unnecessary prescribing. In the UK the Medicines Commission now insists that there is a data sheet published for every drug by the firm that markets it. The data sheet has to be agreed by the Licensing Authority, in consultation

if necessary with the Committee on Safety of Medicines. It is illegal for a firm to promote a drug for any purpose other than those set out in the data sheet.

It is, however, difficult for both the Licensing Authority and the Association of the British Pharmaceutical Industry which has a strict code of advertising to maintain a surveillance of advertisements, and it is almost impossible for them to control what the firms' representatives say to doctors. Some hospitals insist that representatives are only allowed to call on members of the hospital staff, especially the junior medical staff, if they have made an appointment. Some hospitals restrict the generous 'hospitality' which firms extend to the residents' mess. Others although disliking this 'hospitality' believe, as indeed do some of the best firms, that the good sense and competence of young graduates leads them to discredit firms that use such methods.

There has also been concern that many reputable medical journals now depend to an excessive amount on their advertising revenue and accept advertisements which are unworthy of their status. This may be true but an editor is understandably likely to be influenced not only by financial considerations but also by a profound dislike of any censorship or interference with freedom of speech. More disturbing is the recent rash of medical newspapers and magazines sent unsolicited and for no payment to doctors which are a medium both for advertisements and for articles which may be cleverly slanted to encourage the use of drugs.

In recent years firms have made a practice of supporting postgraduate meetings and symposia. It is difficult to draw a line between what is reasonable and what is excessive. There is no doubt that many doctors would not come to postgraduate meetings so readily were it not for the meals and hospitality that are supplied and postgraduate education has benefited from this policy.

Sometimes, however, the hospitality is excessive: free transport to a desirable resort, perhaps abroad, for both the participants and their wives, predominance of papers that are favourable to the products of the firm concerned and gifts that are inappropriately generous are not unknown.

It has been suggested that the DHSS should enter into negotiations with firms with a view to restricting their expenditure on promotion. What is most wanted is that the restrained and reasonable behaviour of the best firms should be accepted by all. This is probably best achieved by persuasion rather than legislation, and would probably be best achieved if doctors evinced more concern about the standards of advertising and refused to be influenced by excessive promotion.

6. *Nationalization of the Pharmaceutical Industry.* Nationalization of the pharmaceutical industry or of part of the industry has been suggested. This suggestion may have a political mileage but it is hard to see that it would bring the price of drugs down substantially. The profit obtained on drugs must usually represent only a fraction of the final prices. The

high standards of purity, the rigorous testing, the demands of the code of good manufacturing insisted on by the Licensing Authority and the nature of research and development, mean amongst other things that this industry employs a higher proportion of university graduates and skilled technicians than any other major industry in the UK. Whether a company is privately owned or is nationalized, producing high quality modern drugs is expensive.

7. *Restrictions on Prescribing.* Numerous proposals have been made for restriction of the drugs or preparations that may be prescribed by doctors. The most recent proposals were outlined in a Bill, Medical Practitioners (Restriction of Right to Prescribe), put before Parliament in May, 1976, which would restrict doctors to simple and innocuous remedies unless they could show that they were regularly attending postgraduate instruction on drugs.

In New Zealand, Australia and Denmark tariff systems have been introduced. Drugs are classified into categories such as 'lifesaving' 'important' and 'others' (Denmark) for which patients pay respectively nothing, a small charge or a large charge. There appear to be no major complaints of inadequate medical treatment from either the public or doctors in countries which have a tariff scheme, but such systems are expensive to administer. There is some argument about the savings achieved but these are probably substantial.

Wade and McDevitt (17) examined the use of the British National Formulary (BNF) by prescribers in Northern Ireland. They found that only about 13-24 per cent of prescriptions were for preparations in the BNF, but that more than 91 per cent of prescriptions could have been written from it, with, in their opinion, no loss to the patient (Table 14.6).

Table 14.6
Analysis of prescriptions in Northern Ireland, 1966

	General sample	*High cost prescriber*	*Low cost prescriber*
Number of prescriptions analysed	695	1558	1294
Prescriptions written for:			
Preparations in BNF	16%	13%	24%
Preparations for which a BNF alternative could have been prescribed	76%	81%	67%
Preparations for which there was no suitable alternative in BNF	5%	2%	6%
Drugs and appliances	4%	4%	4%

At the prices of that time, this would have saved the Northern Ireland Health Service £1 million in a total drug bill of £4.4 million. If such a policy were to be imposed on the whole UK, although it would mean that many fewer preparations of drugs were prescribed than at present, it would seem likely that the prices of those that were prescribed would rise. Although there may be good therapeutic reasons for persuading doctors to prescribe from the BNF it would be wrong to assume it would reduce the drug bill radically, but it would certainly produce a substantial reduction.

In their survey, Wade and McDevitt compared the prescribing of some 'high cost' doctors with 'low cost' doctors. The differences in costs were only marginally due to any difference in the drugs or preparations they prescribed and neither used the BNF very greatly. The different cost was mainly due to the large quantities that the high cost doctor prescribed on each prescription compared with the smaller quantities, usually enough for only a week or ten days which were prescribed by the low cost doctor. If the high cost doctors thought, and some of them appeared to, that by prescribing large amounts they increased the period of time before the patient visited their surgery again it would appear that they were mistaken. In practices of the same size the number of visits from patients for prescriptions were as frequent each month in the high cost as in the low cost practice. In 1954, the New Zealand Health Authority introduced a restriction on the maximum quantity that could be ordered by a doctor at once, and limited this to the amount necessary for 15 days' treatment with the possibility of one repeat. However, the conditions of service of doctors are different in the UK from New Zealand and although doctors should be strongly encouraged to restrict the quantities they prescribe, it would not be easy to supervise a mandatory system and special arrangements would have to be made for a large number of patients with long-term diseases such as diabetes, hypothyroidism, epilepsy or asthma.

A cogent reason for doctors to restrict the quantities they prescribe is the evidence of surveys which show that a large proportion of prescribed medicines are not used by patients. They are kept in the house, sometimes to be used inappropriately for another illness or by another member of the household and sometimes, for they are seldom kept locked in a medicine cupboard, to cause accidental poisoning to a toddler or to be used in self-poisoning by someone in distress or misery. Dunnell and Cartwright (16) in a survey of 1,401 persons, found that 45 per cent of the prescribed medicines in the home had not been used at all in the month before the interview and 25 per cent had not been used in the previous 6 months. Thirty-five per cent of the containers of medicines that had not been used during the previous year were three-quarters full.

A particularly worrying feature of general practice in recent years has been the increasing habit of many doctors to sign repeat prescription forms filled in by a receptionist without the doctor seeing the patient at all.* For a few patients well known to a practice who have a regular need for medicines this may be acceptable. That so many patients now receive repeat prescriptions without question for months or even

*For an interesting review which suggests that this practice is not completely the fault of the doctor, see Balint et al. (18).

years without seeing their doctor, is not only bad medical practice, but is also the cause of a waste of money, for many of these prescriptions are unnecessary.

8. *Financial Incentives to Economize.* Ways of providing doctors with a financial incentive to prescribe economically have not been used since the NHS was established in 1948. But when the National Health Insurance scheme was inaugurated in 1912 arrangements were made so that 2 shillings out of the 9 shilling capitation fee were set aside to form a drug fund. If in any area the cost of drugs fell below 2 shillings per head the difference up to a maximum of 6 pence was added to the remuneration of the doctors in the area. If the cost exceeded 2 shillings per head the pharmacists' accounts were scaled down. This 'floating sixpence' was abolished in 1920. The scheme must have been difficult to administer, and but for the fact that only a limited section of the employed persons in the population were covered by the insurance scheme, it would surely have eventually generated ill-feeling between pharmacists and doctors and between the doctors in an area.

After Wade and McDevitt (17) had completed the survey in Northern Ireland which showed that a saving in pharmaceutical costs might be achieved if doctors prescribed more from the British National Formulary, it was suggested that a sum of £75 per quarter might be paid to all practitioners who could show that 75 per cent of their prescriptions were from the BNF. It is a pity that this suggestion was not accepted for a trial period. It would have shown whether an incentive of this type did or did not achieve what was its main aim: to persuade doctors to think continually of economy in the prescribing of drugs.

9. *Prescribing Budgets.* The idea that doctors should have a drug budget has to date only been considered, and usually rather perfunctorily, in hospitals. With the present restriction of funds in the hospital service it has become increasingly clear that new developments can take place only at the cost of reducing existing commitments and there is now beginning to be discussion, argument and decision about economies. In some hospitals the medical and pharmacy staffs are beginning to examine the use of drugs in their hospital in order to reduce the drug bill (Fig. 14.6). If there is a ward pharmacy service, it is suggested that pharmacists, who are far more knowledgeable than doctors about drug costs, should be requested to keep the medical staff, and particularly the junior medical staff, alerted to the cost of the drugs they prescribe, and especially about the cost of expensive drugs such as antibiotics, corticosteroids and cytotoxic drugs.

The need for the hospital pharmacy to supply drugs to out-patients has also been questioned. This may occasionally be of real importance to patients but it is often no more than a convenience for them. Although its restriction might help a hospital budget and allow a reduction of pharmacy staff, the Health Service would eventually have to meet the

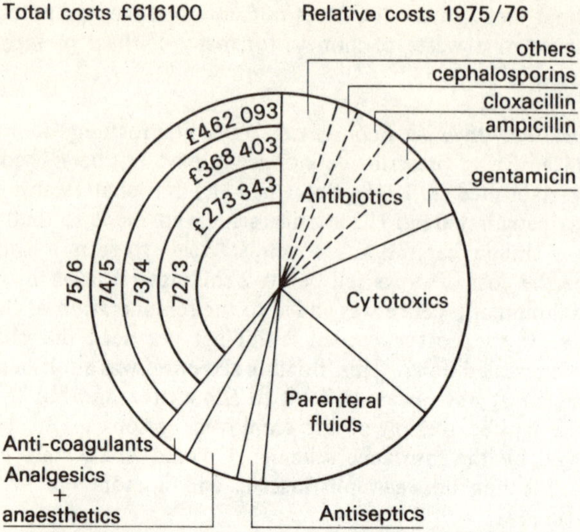

Figure 14.6. Drug costs in a teaching hospital, 1975/76

cost of the drugs after they had been prescribed for the patient by his own doctor. The cost of prescribing outside hospital is greater than the cost in a hospital where the pharmacy is often able to purchase at a discount and has none of the overheads of the pharmacy shop in the High Street (19).

There has to date never been any discussion of the possibility of establishing a prescribing budget for general practitioners. Yet this would seem, on reflection, to be a measure which might effectively reduce the drug bill of the NHS. Each doctor might be given a 'drug allowance' of £400 or £500 per 100 persons on his list to meet the costs of his prescribing. If he prescribed in excess of this, other than in exceptional circumstances, the excess would be met from his practice: if he prescribed within his budget the savings would accrue to his practice profits. In a scheme of this sort there would then be a strong incentive for:

1. The doctor to know the cost of every item he prescribed.
2. The doctor to question the need for every prescription he wrote.
3. The drug industry to be intensely competitive in its drug prices.
4. The drug industry to concentrate its research and development on those products which would be likely to be a real therapeutic advance.

This suggestion is not as revolutionary as it first appears. The principle is already established in a slightly different context where the practitioner is reimbursed for most of his practice expenses with a sum calculated by averaging the costs of a sample of practices. These average costs are obtained by examining the claims submitted from the sample of practices to the Inland Revenue. Practices which keep their costs below this average will gain a profit whereas those where the costs are greater than the average will have a loss.

Conclusion

Modern drugs have brought great benefits to mankind: doctors would not like to practice medicine without penicillin, cortisone or modern vaccines. These benefits would not be available but for the endeavours and skills of the pharmaceutical industry because the production of drugs demands great expertise and rigorous standards of production (20).

There is no doubt, however, that substantial economy in the prescribing of drugs could be achieved: it would not harm patients and it would benefit other sections of the Health Service which are short of money.

What is needed is a change in attitude.

There has, since the beginning of the National Health Service, been a firm and reasonable conviction amongst doctors that the treatment a patient gets should be a matter of decision by a doctor. In their desire to defend this reasonable tenet doctors have resented any criticism of their prescribing, including any criticism of the cost that they incur.

In these times of financial stringency, there is likely to be a reduction in the monies available for the Health Service. It would seem wise for doctors to accept this unpleasant fact and agree to arrangements which reduce the costs of drug prescribing but leave them professional freedom. Unless they do this themselves, restrictions may be imposed upon them by persons who do not understand how important professional freedom is to the health of medicine.

References

1. Ministry of Health (1956). *Report of the Committee of Enquiry into the Cost of the National Health Service* (Guillebaud Report). Cmnd 9663. London, HMSO.
2. Ministry of Health (1959). *Final Report of Committee on Costs of Prescribing* (Hinchcliffe Report). London, HMSO.
3. Ministry of Health (1967). *Committee of Enquiry into the Relationship of the Pharmaceutical Industry with the National Health Service* (Sainsbury Committee). London, HMSO.
4. Department of Health for Scotland (1959). *Report of the Scottish Committee on Prescribing Costs.* Edinburgh, HMSO.
5. Government of Northern Ireland. (1969). *Prescribing and Sickness Benefit Costs in Northern Ireland.* Cmnd 528. Belfast, HMSO.
6. Wade, O.L. (1968). The computer and drug prescribing. In: *Computer in the Service of Medicine.* Ed. McLachlan, G. and Shegog, R.A. London, Oxford University Press.
7. Elmes, P.C., Hood, H. and Wade, O.L. (1976). Prescribing in Northern Ireland. Methods of analysis. *Ulster Medical Journal,* **45**, 56.
8. Elmes, P.C., Hood, H., McMeekin, C. and Wade, O.L. (1976). Prescribing in Northern Ireland. Study No. 1. Sleeping tablets. *Ulster Medical Journal,* **45**, 166.

9. Bergman, U., Elmes, P., Halse, M., Halvorsen, T., Hood, H., Lunde, P.K.M., Sjoquist, F., Wade, O.L. and Westerholm, B. (1975). The measurement of drug consumption. Drugs for diabetes in Northern Ireland, Norway and Sweden. *European Journal of Clinical Pharmacology*, 8, 83.
10. Engels, A. and Siderius, P. (1968). The consumption of drugs. Report of a study 1966-7. Unpublished WHO Working document EURO 3101. Copenhagen.
11. Cochrane, A.L. and Moore, F. (1971). Expected and observed values for the prescription of vitamin B12 in England and Wales. *British Journal of Preventive and Social Medicine*, 25, 147.
12. United States Congress Senate Committee (1963). *Report on Interagency Coordination in Drug Research and Regulation.* Washington DC, Government Printing Office.
13. Cooper, J.D. (Editor) (1970). *The Economics of Drug Innovation*, p. 133. Washington, American University.
14. Fattorusso, V. (1976). Eighth Assembly of the IFPMA, London, 17-18 June. *ABPI News*, No. 162.
15. Abel-Smith, B. (1976). *Value for Money in the Health Services.* Heinemann. London.
16. Dunnell, K. and Cartwright, A. (1972). *Medicine Takers, Prescribers and Hoarders.* London, Routledge & Kegan Paul.
17. Wade, O.L. and McDevitt, G.D. (1966). Prescribing and the British National Formulary. *British Medical Journal*, 2, 635.
18. Balint, M., Hunt, I., Joyce, D., Marinker, M. and Woodcock, J. (1970). *Treatment or Diagnosis. A study of repeat prescriptions in general practice.* London, Tavistock.
19. Opit, L.J. and Farmer, R.D.T. (1974). Cost of dispensing in the pharmaceutical services. *Lancet*, i, 160.
20. Department of Health and Social Security (1976). *Guide to Good Manufacturing Practice.* London, HMSO.

15

Use and Misuse of Drugs in the Treatment of the Chronic Psychoses

Henry R. Rollin

'It may seem a strange principle to enunciate as the very first requirement in a hospital that it should do the sick no harm.'

Florence Nightingale, 1859

Psychiatrists who have survived three or four decades of work in mental hospitals have become inured to therapeutic miracles. They have witnessed the much heralded appearance (and ignominious disappearance) of a variety of 'miracles', such as deep insulin therapy and, the most disastrous of them all, prefrontal leucotomy 1950s style. For each and every one of the therapies, the claim was made that it could cure, or at any rate, ameliorate, schizophrenia – a shorthand term for a group of similar, but by no means identical, mental illnesses, illnesses which will remain for the foreseeable future one of psychiatry's major preoccupations.

The introduction of the psychotropic drugs was heralded as yet another miracle. Such is the power of suggestion brought about by acres of important papers in important journals by important people reinforced by the persuaders, hidden and otherwise, of the drug manufacturers, that this time the miracle was believed to be 'for real'. But then, as the initial euphoria wore off a more critical examination of the newest of the Emperor's new clothes became possible. Sadly, they were less than perfect. The major imperfections seemed to be in relation to those patients who remained continuously or intermittently under our scrutiny for long periods; i.e. those who have been chosen to be called 'chronic psychotics'. Almost daily contact with a particular group of such patients brought the realization that, in spite of psychotropic drugs, the natural history of the illness was persisted in. There was, that is, in most cases, an inexorable and irreversible deterioration to be seen in the whole personality, accompanied sometimes by periods of remission alternating with relapses in which bouts of excitement occasioning serious behaviour disturbance occurred. The course of the illness was graphically described years ago by Professor Desmond Curran as a switchback going downhill. The description still applies. At this juncture a plea must be made for the demolition of the myth of the 'burnt-out schizophrenic'. Experience has shown that it is advisable always to be on guard against a sudden rekindling of the embers of a psychosis which would appear to be dead.

A further observation of equal importance was that attempts to arrest this built-in deterioration with potent drugs impose side-effects – side-effects which were almost as painful to witness as they must have been to those who suffered them. Reference is made, of course, to a variety of extrapyramidal reactions including dryness of mouth, dyskinesia, akathisia, restlessness and, on occasion, irreversible tardive dyskinesia.

It seemed obvious that if no benefit accrued – indeed, if positive ill-effects were being inflicted – then some patients might be better off without drugs. But which? The only way to attempt to find out, it appeared, was to remove all such drugs from a group of patients living under more-or-less identical conditions.

Ward 14 at Horton Hospital seemed to offer the best opportunity for such an experiment. It is a large ward divided into dormitory accommodation at one side, and dining and day accommodation on the other. It had been upgraded, and within limits is comfortable enough. The ward was supervised during the day by one charge nurse with one part-time orderly. At night the ward was visited by a patrol nurse only. Medically it had come under the author's day-to-day supervision.

In view of the very light nursing cover, episodes of prolonged seriously disturbed behaviour could not be tolerated and patients had of necessity to be transferred temporarily or even permanently to more appropriate wards.

However, what made Ward 14 suitable for an experiment in drug withdrawal was that, in relation to other wards in the hospital, it had a fairly static population of males, and that clinically it was reasonably homogeneous. It was, in old terminology, a 'workers ward for chronics' – a blunt but not inappropriate description.

On the 31st December 1967 there were 60 patients in the ward, 53 of whom were receiving medication. The latter were to be the subjects of the experiment and what follows applies exclusively to them.

Demographic Data

Age. The age range was from 27 to 64, distributed as shown in Table 15.1.

The mean age is 47.7 years and it is evident that the majority (87 per cent) were over 40 years of age.

Country of Birth. Twenty-nine (55 per cent) were born in the UK; 9 (17 per cent) were born in Eire, 4 (7.5 per cent) in Poland, 2 in India and the

Table 15.1
Age of patients on 31.12.67

Age group	*No. of patients*
20-29	3
30-39	4
40-49	23
50-59	19
60-69	4
Total	53

rest made up by single representatives from the West Indies, Czechoslovakia, Switzerland, Cyprus, the Ukraine, Latvia, Germany, Russia and Egypt.

The polyglot collection in the ward reflects, of course, the make-up of our then catchment area, which was largely the old borough of Paddington, London.

Marital Status. Of the 53 patients, 39 (74 per cent) were single, 5 were separated and 1 had been divorced. The very high percentage of single (never married) is in accord with other studies of the marital status of schizophrenics.

Contact with Families and the Outside World. Contact with either relatives or other persons in the outside world can be measured by a variety of indices. In the case of our 53 patients, I chose to measure it by week-end leave spent at their parental or marital home or with friends, by visits of family or friends to the hospital and by postal contact. Only 4 patients paid regular week-end visits to their homes and 3 others did so only very occasionally. Only 13 of the 53 were ever visited – some weekly, others fortnightly or less frequently; and the number who received letters, parcels and the like was limited to a mere 15.

The social picture is, therefore, of a group of isolated, forgotten men for whom the hospital was a home, or, more exactly, an asylum in the best use of the term. Some might readily have left hospital if 'community care' had real meaning and they had 'some place to go'.

Clinical Data

Diagnosis. As might have been expected, the overwhelming majority of the patients (i.e. 46; 87 per cent) suffered from schizophrenia. The remaining comprised 3 manic-depressives, a demented GPI, an inadequate personality, a schizo-affective psychotic and an (?) epileptic with a superimposed paranoid psychosis who had had no recorded fits for years.

Chronicity. The chronicity of the psychoses can be measured by the number of admissions to Horton and other mental hospitals in conjunction with the length of time spent in them in the aggregate. The difficulty in accumulating such data is notorious and the results must, therefore, be considered as minimal. Nevertheless, the data are impressive.

Table 15.2
Number of admissions to mental hospitals

No. of admissions	*No. of cases*
1	12
2	16
3	13
4	5
5	1
9	3
10	1
11	1
12	1
Total	53 (mean 3.1)

The range in the number of admissions is, therefore, from 1 to 12 (mean 13.1), with an overwhelming preponderance of more than one admission.

Table 15.3
Duration of the psychoses

Period in years	*No. of cases*
0-5	6
5-10	8
10-15	10
15-20	21
20-25	3
25-30	3
30+	2
Total	53 (mean 16.6 years)

The range is thus from less than 5 years to over 30 years (mean 16.6 years).

Taking Tables 15.2 and 15.3 together the evidence is indisputable: the patients concerned were suffering, in the vast majority of cases, from a severe, chronic psychosis; namely, schizophrenia.

Previous Physical Treatment. The chronicity of the psychoses together with the age of most of the patients made it likely that more than less would have been exposed to one or more forms of physical treatment in the past in accordance, that is, with the fashion of the time. This proved to be the case.

The results of the analyses are shown in Table 15.4. In fact, in only 3 cases had no previous treatment been administered. It is evident that the failure to arrest the natural history of the psychoses was not for want of trying.

Table 15.4
Previous physical treatments

A. Leucotomy	5
B. Deep insulin therapy	19
C. ECG	49

Combination of previous physical treatment

A (alone)	1	B (alone)	—
A + B	—	B + C	17
A + C	2	C (alone)	27
		A + B + C	2

Current Treatment on 31.12.67. It is an index of the tremendous increase in the use of psychotropic drugs in the 1960s – chlorpromazine (Largactil), trifluoperazine (Stelazine), promazine (Sparine) and perphenazine (Fentazin) – that 51 of the 53 patients were on varying doses of one or the other drugs, and in some instances had been on them for a matter of years.

It is noteworthy that on 31.12.67, 32 were receiving some form of night sedation, 18 of whom were on amylobarbitone sodium (Sodium Amytal) 400 mg every night. The others were on methaqualone (Mandrax). The 2 patients not receiving psychotropic drugs were on night sedation only.

Method. The method was simple in the extreme, if seemingly heroic. In consultation with the nursing staff, and such a step could not have been even contemplated without their full co-operation, it was agreed to stop all drugs in all 53 cases as from midnight on 31.12.67. The proscription would, therefore, apply not only to psychotropic drugs, but night sedatives and the anticonvulsive drug primidone (Mysoline) in the one very doubtful case of epilepsy. Initially in all cases of night sedation placebo drugs were to be substituted. It was further agreed that in no case would the experiment preclude discharge or 'promotion' to other wards. Neither would it prevent transfer to other wards for the usual administrative reasons; nor, of course, in the event of outbursts of disturbed behaviour which could not be tolerated in a ward as lightly staffed as Ward 14, would it prevent transfer to a more appropriate ward temporarily, or, if need be, permanently. And, most importantly, if it was considered in the best interests of the patient that drugs should be restored, this would be done. The experiment was to last for one year; i.e. until 31.12.68 in the first instance. A follow-up would be extended for as long as possible thereafter.

Results. These were awaited with not a little apprehension. There was a general feeling that what was about to be done amounted to something approaching sacrilege and that the displeasure of those gods who were offended would be manifested one way or another. In actual fact the skies did not fall: the ward was not beset with plague or pestilence. The only complaint was that of sleeplessness on the part of 8 patients who for long periods had been accustomed to receiving Sodium Amytal 400 mg nightly. It was evident as the sleeplessness persisted that they had become drug-dependent. In 5 of the 8 night sedation had to be restored but they seemed content with 200 mg of the drug and a placebo tablet. In the case of those patients who had been on psychotropic drugs precisely nothing happened initially except that some side-effects began to evaporate. However, as time went on symptoms erupted which in all cases could be attributable to the natural history of the mental illness and had to be dealt with in a variety of ways.

Results of Experiment

The basic disposal of the patients on 31.12.68 is shown in Table 15.5.

Table 15.5
Disposal of patients until 31.12.68

Discharges	4
Permanent transfers to other wards	13
Temporary transfers to other wards	9
Retained on Ward 14. Drugs resumed	3
Retained on Ward 14. All drugs omitted	24
Total	53

NB. On 31.12.74, that is after a follow-up of 7 years, 11 of the original population were still on Ward 14 and had had no psychotropic drugs.

Discharges. Four patients were discharged: 1 by repatriation and 3 by absconding.

Permanent Transfers. Thirteen patients were transferred permanently to other wards. Six were transferred for administrative reasons. Seven patients were transferred because their persistent disturbed behaviour made their retention on Ward 14 impossible: 3 were persistent absconders and had had to be repeatedly returned by the police; 1 was a dangerous fire-raiser and 1 needed closer supervision to guarantee his personal hygiene; 2 were too aggressive to be contained on the ward. All 7 went to a locked ward. It is most important to note that all these patients had exhibited similar disturbed behaviour when on psychotropic drugs.

Temporary Transfers. Nine patients were temporarily transferred to a locked ward during periods of disturbed behaviour. In most instances the period of transfer was for no more than 14 days. Again, all these patients had had recorded episodes of similar behaviour disturbances when on psychotropic drugs.

Retained on Ward 14, but Drugs Resumed. Three patients became disturbed, but not so gravely as to necessitate transfer to locked wards. However, the reintroduction of drugs was considered necessary to allow them to remain on Ward 14. Here again, episodes of disturbance had been noted in the past when they had been on psychotropic drugs.

Retained on Ward 14, Without Drugs. Of special importance were the 24 (45 per cent) who were maintained on Ward 14 without psychotropic drugs for the entire year, all of whom had been on them at the outset of the experiment. Enquiries were made from the heads of utility and occupational departments in which some of the patients worked. In several instances they commented that the patients were more 'with-it', or that they appeared less tired. It could be fairly said, therefore, that in these 24 patients at least there was no call for psychotropic drugs to be administered on a permanent basis.

Followed-up for 7 Years. In the follow-up of these 24 patients for 7 years (that is, until 31.12.74), 2 had died, 5 had been transferred to other wards for a variety of reasons, and 2 had been discharged. Of the 15 remaining on Ward 14, 4 had had drugs restored for limited periods of time during exacerbations of their chronic psychosis; one, in fact, on 24.12.74, a few days before the end of the follow-up. He had gone home for Christmas leave, as he had done regularly at week-ends over the years, but this time for no apparent reason he had attacked his aged mother and had to be returned immediately to the hospital – further evidence, if such be needed, of the doubtful validity of the concept of the 'burnt-out schizophrenic'. Eleven (21 per cent) patients of the original population had, therefore, remained completely off drugs for 7 years.

Financial Saving. Of importance, too, in these days of economic stringency is the saving in the cost of the drugs omitted, amounting, in the course of 1968 alone, to £800 approximately. The saving at today's prices would be considerably more.

Conclusions

The experiment described is admittedly an exercise in pragmatism. The author had long suspected that in those patients deliberately described as suffering from chronic psychoses – in the overwhelming majority of cases, chronic schizophrenia – no treatment so far devised has succeeded in arresting the natural history of the disease. Experience has shown that this pessimistic prognosis, in spite of claims to the contrary, obtains just as much in chronic psychotics who have been maintained on psychotropic drugs for long periods of time. The fact that the total withdrawal of the drugs produced no deleterious effects, but, on the contrary, proved beneficial in a number of cases, would also support this conclusion – a conclusion reached by Hughes and Crawford Little (1), Andrews, Hall and Smith (2), and Fottrell and Sheikh (3).

Nevertheless, it would be absurd to maintain that there is no place for psychotropic drugs in the treatment of the chronic psychoses. Their use in acute exacerbations of the illnesses has been described. The plea that is fervently made in the prescription of these very potent and potentially dangerous drugs is for constant vigilance. To expose our patients to them unnecessarily would be to offend against the prayer of Florence Nightingale – that a hospital should do the sick no harm.

References

1. Hughes, J.S. and Crawford Little, J. (1967). An appraisal of the continuing practice of prescribing tranquillising drugs for long-stay psychiatric patients. *British Journal of Psychiatry*, **113**, 867.
2. Andrews, P., Hall, J.N. and Smith, R.P. (1976). A controlled trial of phenothiazine withdrawal in chronic schizophrenic patients. *British Journal of Psychiatry*, **128**, 451.
3. Fottrell, E. and Sheikh, M. (1976). Long-stay patients with long-stay drugs. A case for review: a cause for concern. *Lancet*, **i**, 81.

16

Price Sensitivity of General Practitioners

W. Duncan Reekie

To most observers the pharmaceutical industry is one in which price competition is conspicuous by its absence. Instead, the main forms of interfirm rivalry are those of promotion and product quality differentiation.

This view complies closely with the reported pattern of frequent product innovation, associated high promotion expenditures and infrequent price alterations of existing products. No one, however, as far as I know, has examined in detail the implications of a lack of price competition for the pricing behaviour to be expected from new medicinal products; nor the degree of correspondence between the behaviour so implied and the observable price/market performance pattern of such innovations. These two tasks will be undertaken in Sections I and II respectively of this paper. Section III will summarize the conclusions and discuss some possible public policy implications which arise and which would affect the industry's relationship with the National Health Service.

I The Received View

Medicines are a necessity and as such an increase in price will drive few people from the market nor will a fall attract many in. This necessity effect which results in demand inelasticity is reinforced by the fact that the actual selection of the product is made by a third party, the doctor, not the patient or final consumer and, at least in the UK, payment is made by a fourth party to the transaction, the National Health Service. Cooper (1) has stated that 'demand responds to the incidence of sickness, the quality of therapy available to treat it, and to sales promotion, but very little else'. In other words, the industry may be close to the Galbraithian situation where the firm 'controls the prices at which it sells and takes steps to insure that the public, other producers, or the state take the planned quantities at these prices' (2).

Secondly, firms adjust their prices according to the actions of those rivals whose products are close substitutes. In pharmaceuticals this condition exists within the highly concentrated therapeutic submarkets,* between which cross-elasticity of demand is low. In accordance with at least some oligopoly theories, price competition should, therefore, not be expected. Prices will tend to be rigid, and that at a high level. Comanor (3) adheres to this view and suggests that the consequent existence of monopoly profits reduces the pressures on drug firms to lower costs. Lower costs, he argues, could permit the charging of lower prices, but, given inelastic demand and oligopolistic uncertainties, this would not lead to sufficiently attractive increases in revenues. The use of price as an important competitive tool is, consequently, unlikely.

Thirdly the prices of existing pharmaceutical products are rarely altered (1) and when product duplication occurs price equivalence is frequently the case (4).

The Monopolies Commission (5) would view the first two of these points (inelastic demand and high concentration levels) as necessary (although not sufficient) conditions from which to predict the probable absence of price competition in an industry. In which case the third point (stable, parallel prices) could be deduced to be the outcome of collusive, monopolistic price leadership and not that of competitive forces.

The Sainsbury Committee (6), in a specific study of the pharmaceutical industry, concluded that they 'did not gain the impression that there was any significant degree of price competition in medical specialty products'. This conclusion was arrived at after the Committee had asked firms how prices were determined. Some said they considered the prices of alternatives, others that they aimed to obtain a required rate of return on investment and others that they tried to recover cost in a given period. These objectives need not be incompatible, but the latter two in particular could appear to depend on rule of thumb pricing tools. Many writers have argued persuasively that the use of such rules helps eliminate oligopolistic uncertainties and increases industry discipline in loose-knit cartels.† In the USA the Congressional Committee chaired by Senator Kefauver came to similar conclusions in its report

*That is, groupings of medicines such as analgesics, anaesthetics, antibiotics, anticoagulants, etc.

†An excellent survey of this literature is given by F.M. Scherer (7).

in 1961, 'Administered Prices: Drugs'.*

If all of this is true, if pharmaceutical firms are selling their products to price-insensitive consumers (i.e. doctors), and if monopolistic price leadership is the norm, what characteristics can be expected to emerge from the pricing patterns of innovations? For the empirical tests of Section II, the following differences between the implications of a market with collusive suppliers and price-inelastic consumers on the one hand, and a market with competing suppliers and price-sensitive consumers on the other will be used.

1. The simplest theories of demand elasticity and collusion are silent on innovation. They are restricted to the two dimensions of price and quantity. Consequently no guidance is given as to the level at which the price of an innovation will be pitched. If the collusion is simply extended to embrace innovation then the price selected will be at or near to the prices of existing products. More realistically, firms may regard innovations as 'focal points' in decision making. Prices would then be pitched above existing levels and other sellers would always expect this. Uncertainty about price changes would be reduced, other firms would raise their prices, probably with the aid of some real or illusory product differentiation of their own, and the behaviour pattern of price co-ordination would be strengthened. This picture of generally rising prices is more in line with the facts than that of a consistent overall pharmaceutical price level over time. However, no indication of *what* price increase should be expected from an innovation can be inferred from this discussion. If the degree of price co-ordination is very strong then presumably a similar absolute or relative change will occur on each occasion on which an innovation 'focal point' is reached. If it is weaker then some more-or-less random distribution of price increases would be expected.

On the other hand, if the market is composed of competing suppliers, if collusion is weak or non-existent, and if the assumption that doctors are non-price sensitive is also relaxed then a somewhat different picture emerges. Firms can then be expected to price major breakthroughs well above the cost of previous inferior treatments. Minor variants, on the other hand, would be priced below competitors so as to give them some promotional advantage.

*The nature of official views about the industry's pricing behaviour can also be inferred from specific cases. In 1962, the Minister of Health, Mr Enoch Powell, partially removed patent protection from Pfizer's then leading brand Terramycin by invoking Section 46 of the Patents Act. This was a deliberate attempt to impose price pressures on the company which the market was failing to do. In 1973 the Monopolies Commission condemned Roche Products Ltd for charging prices for its two drugs Librium and Valium which were 'manifestly too high'. The Commission did report that their daily dosage costs were 'amongst the lowest when compared with competitive products' but then went on to claim that there was a *'virtual absence of price competition'* (emphasis added) (8).

2. The parallel price/inelastic demand model suggests that prices will be pitched high and remain stable. This is the view adopted, for example, by Lall who states that 'the pricing policies of the large drug firms are based on purely monopolistic principles ... rather than on the socially responsible one of lowering them after recovering research costs' (9). The effectively competitive model, however, predicts that the price level of innovations will vary not only with the degree of rivalry from existing substitutes but also with that from anticipated competition. Thus major breakthroughs will tend to be reduced in price over time as new competition becomes more and more likely; or, more dramatically, even a major breakthrough will be priced low if the firm feels its competitive edge will be short lived due to the imminent advent of another competing innovation. In other words, to obtain a toehold in the market for any length of time a low price is necessary to generate prescriber goodwill.

New pharmaceuticals, then, can be introduced at a high price designed to extract the highest possible revenue when demand (for these products) is relatively inelastic, and thereafter gradually reduced in price through the product life cycle. A rationale for this policy, what Joel Dean (10) called 'skimming pricing', is easy to give. First, a high initial cash flow is required to repay as rapidly as possible the innovative outlays of the firm; secondly, as time passes price sensitivity increases as the government exerts pressure through the Voluntary Price Regulation Scheme (VPRS) on the one hand, and competitors retaliate with similarly priced, but equally or possibly more advanced innovations of their own; finally, lower priced rivals will begin to appear as patent expiry approaches or Section 41 (the compulsory licensing provision of the Patents Act) is invoked. (There is the additional argument, in some markets such as antibiotics where scale economies are important, that a high price is required to cover relatively high unit production costs when and if output is still low.)

The alternative extreme is a policy of 'penetration pricing'. This occurs where prices are set at a relatively low level immediately on market launch. It may be adopted when the product represents only a minor departure from those previously available and so is unable to command a substantial premium over existing, not dissimilar, alternatives. It may also be used as a discouraging 'keep out' policy in anticipation of new and rival entrants.

Between these two extremes there will, of course, be a continuum of possible relative price levels. I have shown elsewhere (11) how price discrimination over time (skimming) can be perfectly justifiable in welfare terms. Pharmaceuticals have very low marginal costs. Skimming prices enable firms to appropriate consumers' surplus to themselves by charging the successive reservation prices and so provide revenue to pay for research and development investment costs (rather on the lines of the perfectly discriminating monopolist who finds he *can* justify the building of Dupuit's bridge).

3. The final contrasting implication is that if doctors are price insensitive then, even if price differentials exist, there will be little variation in the market performance of similar products. Not only will the industry demand curve be inelastic, but the demand curve for individual products will also be inelastic. This is the view, for example, of Cooper (12) who alleges that 'despite all evidence to the contrary, many men in the industry are still of the opinion that there is a commercial advantage to be gained from cutting prices ... (this) in the face of facts consistently disproving their expectations'.*

Contrariwise, if prescribers are price sensitive, higher priced products will not be as commercially successful as lower priced ones.

II The Empirical Study

The Sample. All new chemical entities introduced on to the UK market between 1962 and 1970 were identified. (Thus possibly significant innovations resulting from combinations or representations of existing compounds were ignored.) The list was abridged by restricting it to entities launched in therapeutic submarkets which accounted for at least 1 per cent of NHS sales in any one of the relevant years. The resulting sample totalled 125 compounds which were sold in the 35 submarkets (out of a possible 80 or so) which accounted, in 1973, for 84.2 per cent of all NHS sales.

The sample of compounds was drawn from an original list of 470 entities launched on to all world markets between 1958 and 1970 and compiled for NEDO's study of 'Innovative Activity in the Pharmaceutical Industry' (13). The list was abbreviated when non-UK launches were excluded. Launches in the UK from 1958 to 1961 were also excluded because basic price and sales data relating to the products were not available in a satisfactory form. Trivial submarkets which in no year achieved 1 per cent of NHS sales were excluded since it was judged that the effort involved in data processing in these markets would far outweigh the benefits to be gained from any additional informational output they might provide. (The final lists of product names and of therapeutic markets are available on request.)

The 125 entities were ranked on a '1' to '5' scale during the NEDO study by pharmacological or clinical experts in the relevant discipline. Table 16.1 provides the definitions of the five rankings for therapeutic value. The assessments were made in the light of the historical situation at the actual date of launch. Thus a fundamental advance at its time of

*Cooper makes this point after studying the price history of a small number of products. An alternative interpretation of his results is that managers will be unaware of the precise price level at which demand becomes relatively inelastic. As a consequence price reductions may well be justified, but because of their trial and error nature may go beyond the optimum point.

Table 16.1
Definitions for five rankings of 'therapeutic value'

1. Fundamental new medicine, of major clinical significance.
2. Important new medicine, offering substantial advantages for a majority of patients.
3. Useful new medicine, offering advantages for a minority of patients.
4. New medicine offering only marginal advantages over previously available therapies.
5. New medicine offering little or no advantage over previously available therapies.

introduction would be ranked '1' even if it was quickly superseded. 'Advantages' included reduction in side-effects as well as improved therapeutic response.

The Variables. The two main economic variables examined were price and market performance. In addition to these, information was assembled relating to whether or not a launch was rapidly succeeded by another new product introduction.

Price must clearly relate to treatment costs and not to volume of tablets, capsules or whatever. In this study price was measured by daily dosage cost. This was obtained in the following manner. The Medical Data Index (published by Intercontinental Medical Statistics) provides a frequency distribution of the daily prescribed dosage of each drug by general practitioners. The modal daily dosage and its form of presentation were selected as 'representative' for the product in question. Thus, for example, it may be discovered that product 'X' is most 'typically' prescribed in 250 mg capsule form on a four times daily basis. This information was then compared with the container price data provided in the British Pharmaceutical Index (also published by IMS). The modal container size sold to pharmacists was selected as 'representative' for the product and the price abstracted accordingly. Thus 250 mg capsules of product 'X' might be sold in containers of 100, 500 or 1000 capsules. Generally the larger the container the lower is the price. The container which had the largest financial volume of sales was regarded as the modal container. The appropriate price per capsule for product 'X' could then easily be obtained, and, multiplied by 4, be transformed into the relevant daily dosage cost.

Four indices of relative price were then constructed for each of the 125 innovations:

I. The ratio of innovation price to the simple arithmetic average of the prices of the leading three products in the relevant therapeutic submarket in the year of launch.

II. The ratio of innovation price to the weighted average of the prices of the leading three products. The weights used were the market shares of the top three products.

III. As I, using the prices of the top five products.

IV. As II, using the prices of the leading five products.

Only in the case of corticosteroid creams and ointments was this formulation departed from. There, 'price' could not refer to average daily dosage cost. The straightforward price per gram of ointment was used. This, of course, is a perfectly admissible approach with such a presentation. Usage depends on patient habit and on skin area to be covered. Price per gram (of ointment, *not* active ingredient) is consequently satisfactory for the purposes of 'like-with-like' comparisons. The price of the most commonly sold pack was used to obtain the price per gram.

The price of the innovation was the price in the launch year, year 't'. On a very few occasions this price was changed by the firm, in year 't' itself or in 't + 1' or 't + 2'. Where this occurred, a weighted average price was calculated using market shares for weights.

For all products, including the more voluminous list of comparative products, when price changes occurred during a year, the price deemed to rule for that calendar year was the price which ruled for longer than 6 months plus 1 day.

Market success was measured by two alternative criteria:

A. Share achieved of the relevant submarket in the first two calendar years of product life (i.e. almost always years t + 1 and t + 2).

B. As A, but for the first three years.

Sales data and market share information were consequently abstracted from the British Pharmaceutical Index from 1962 through to 1972.

The Empirical Findings. Table 16.2 provides frequency distributions for the first of the four indices of relative price analysed by therapeutic rank*. *Approximately one-third of all innovations were introduced at lower prices than the leading available substitutes.* (The ratio of innovation price to existing products' prices was less than unity.) From this (penetration) extreme, *the whole continuum of pricing policies is followed* right through to skimming price levels where the innovations were intro-

Table 16.2
Frequency distributions of relative innovative prices
(products analysed by therapeutic value)

Rank	*Nos.*	*>4.0-4.0*	*<4.0-2.0*	*<2.0-1.33*	*<1.33-1.0*	*<1.0*
1	19	3	9	3	2	2
2	23	2	10	3	1	7
3	22	1	6	7	2	6
4	28	3	1	7	6	11
5	33	0	4	7	7	15
	125	9	30	27	18	41

*Irrespective of which index is used, the results are virtually identical.

duced at prices which were a multiple of four or more times as great as that of existing market leaders. Finally, a cursory inspection of the data seems to indicate that the majority of the observations tend to lie either to the top and left of the tables or to the bottom and right. In other words, *high therapeutic value innovations tend to be priced more highly than do those with minimal or zero advantages over existing therapies.*

This latter conclusion is statistically, as well as economically, significant. The calculated chi-squared value is 31.61 (compared with a value of 26.296 at the 5 per cent level of significance). The contingency coefficient is 0.45 (while a 5 x 5 table has a maximum contingency coefficient value of 0.894).

What we have not yet shown is whether a high price, once set, is more likely to fall, rise or remain the same. This could be difficult to illustrate empirically for two reasons. First, a stable monetary price in inflationary conditions is, in fact, a falling price. Secondly, most drugs do have stable prices over lengthy periods of time. Table 16.3, however, using the same

Table 16.3
Frequency distributions of year-by-year price changes, 1962-1973 (all innovations analysed by relative price at date of launch)

	Relative price									
	>4.0-4.0		*<4.0-2.0*		*<2.0-1.33*		*<1.33-1.0*		*<1.0*	
	No.	*%*	*No.*	*%*	*No.*	*%*	*No.*	*%*	*No.*	*%*
Possible	53	100.0	213	100.0	142	100.0	126	100.0	312	100.0
Falls	9	17.0	23	10.8	17	12.0	7	5.5	34	10.9
Rises	2	3.8	14	26.4	9	6.3	8	6.3	27	8.7
Ratio of falls to rises	4.5		1.6		1.9		0.9		1.3	

	>4.0-1.33	*<1.33-<1.0*
Possible	408	438
Falls	49	41
Rises	25	35
Ratio of falls to rises	2.0	1.2

frequency classifications and price index as Table 16.2, does show that initially more expensive products were more likely to be reduced in price than products priced at relatively lower levels: 17 per cent of the costliest products fell in price between 1962 and 1973; 10.8 per cent and 12 per cent respectively of products in the next two most expensive classes experienced price reductions; and 5.5 per cent of innovations in the < 1.33-1.0 class fell in price. The 10.9 per cent of possible price changes which were falls observed in the cheapest classification is less understandable. They may represent 'last throws' to purchase prescriber goodwill with products already known to be commercial failures. Study of individual products is probably necessary to ascertain the true reason. Conversely, given a rising general price level, if penetration and skimming policies are being pursued then one would expect more price rises at the penetration end of the spectrum than at the skimming end. Products priced at low penetration level would tend to have their prices raised in line with the overall price level, thus maintaining a low price. Products priced at a high skimming level would be more likely to have their monetary prices held steady, thus being subject to real price reductions. Table 16.3 provides support for this view. The data indicate that 8.7 per cent of the cheapest products rose in price compared with 3.8 per cent of the dearest. This is not a substantial differential, but its contribution to the overall importance of Table 16.3 is highlighted by the summary ratios of falls to rises for 'expensive' and 'cheap' innovations (i.e. the >4.0-1.33 and <1.33-<1.0 categories respectively).*

Price falls in both categories were more common than price rises, but initially cheaper products were relatively more likely to be raised in price while more expensive products were both absolutely and relatively more likely to be lowered in price.

Table 16.4 provides a frequency distribution for market performance index A, analysed by therapeutic rank.† *A substantial minority of innovations perform very poorly.* (They fail to achieve a cumulative market

Table 16.4
Frequency distribution of market performance (products analysed by therapeutic value)

Rank	*Nos.*	*0-5%*	*>5%-10%*	*>10%-20%*	*>20%*
1	19	6	1	4	8
2	23	9	2	3	9
3	22	4	5	4	9
4	28	15	9	2	2
5	33	23	5	5	0
	125	57	22	18	28

share of 5 per cent after two years, i.e. 2.5 per cent in an average year.) Visual inspection also indicates that most minor innovations perform poorly (many observations 'cluster' in the bottom left-hand corner of Table 16.4), *while major innovations are much more likely to be commercially successful* (a less clear-cut but still apparent 'clustering' takes place in the top right-hand corner of Table 16.4). Statistical support for these conclusions is given by calculating chi-squared, which, at 37.4, is well above the 26.22 value it attains at the 1 per cent significance level.

* Similar results were obtained from the use of the other price indices.

† A comparable picture is obtained using index B.

These results (and also those obtained using the alternative price and performance indices) are summarized in Table 16.5. There the sample

Table 16.5
Average numbers of innovations classed as 'successes' and 'failures', grouped by 'high' and 'low' prices

	High price	*Low price*
'Major' innovations		
Successes	19.6	26.0
Failures	8.9	9.7
'Minor' innovations		
Successes	5.5	19.5
Failures	3.5	32.5

See main text for definitions of 'major' and 'minor' innovations; 'high' and 'low' prices; and 'successes' and 'failures'.

has been subdivided into 64 'major' innovations which were awarded a rank of 1, 2 or 3 and the 61 'minor' innovations which were regarded as having only marginal or no advantages over existing therapies (ranks 4 and 5). The product data were then cross-classified 'High' and 'Low' priced and as 'Successes' or 'Failures'. The boundaries for these categories were the 2.0 price ratio and above for 'High' priced products; and over 5 per cent and 7.5 per cent (for performance variables A and B respectively) for 'Successful' products. Since Table 16.5 is an average of eight similar tables (four for each 'price' yardstick, and two of each of these for the 'performance' criteria), it is inevitable that the figures in the cells usually take on fractional values. Given the close relationships observed between price indices I-IV and performance indicators A and B, however, the averaging process adopted here will not distort the results in any significant manner. The benefit derived from so averaging the results is the not unimportant one that the visual presentation of the data is simplified. Minor eccentricities which appear if any one pair of indices is used in isolation are smoothed away and inferences are consequently easier to make.

The boundaries, of course, are essentially arbitrary, as was the averaging procedure. Disaggregation of the data and variation in the cut-off points would not, however, alter the picture.

Figure 16.1 is constructed from the data in Table 16.5, but the figures for the innovative ranks 1 to 5 have first been disaggregated. What implications can be drawn from this diagram? There is little need to apply sophisticated statistical testing to the figures. Indeed the nature and style of presentation of the information, plus the smallness of sample size, probably preclude this. It is possibly best to let the data speak for themselves.

1. Only innovations of major therapeutic value are likely to be both highly priced and successful (top and bottom right quadrants).

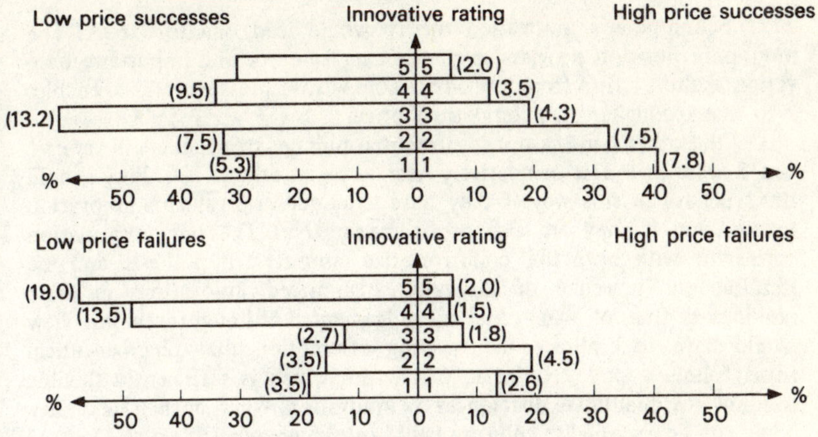

Figure 16.1 Market success and relative price (percentage of products by therapeutic innovative rank). Number of products given in parentheses.

2. Major innovations are more likely to be priced at skimming levels than are minor ones (top right quadrant).

3. Penetration pricing policies are more likely to be adopted for 'useful minority' innovations (rank 3) than they are for 'fundamental' or 'important majority' innovations (ranks 1 and 2). This is the case in relative terms, as comparison of the 'stepped' effect and the 'inverse stepped' effect of ranks 1-3 in the two top quadrants shows. It is also true absolutely. The ratios of numbers of new products introduced in the two quadrants in these ranks fell into the pattern 7.8:5.3 > 7.5:7.5 > 4.3:13.2.

4. When minor innovations (ranks 4 and 5) are successful, they are generally introduced at a low price level (top two quadrants).

5. Even a low price cannot prevent the majority of 'marginal' advances (rank 4) from being failures. This is even more true of near-identical (rank 5) products (bottom left quadrant).

6. Major innovations (ranks 1-3) are unlikely to be launched at a low price level and fail to make a market impact (top and bottom left quadrants).

7. Firms avoid pricing low value innovations (ranks 4 and 5) at high price levels (bottom and top right quadrants).

8. There is weak evidence that high-priced failures occur more frequently in ranks 1 and 2 than in ranks 3, 4 and 5 (bottom right quadrant).

The new products which are most obviously priced at a high, skimming, level fall into therapeutic ranks 1 and 2. Most others are priced, relatively speaking, at or near to the prices of existing substitutes. Price/marginal cost ratios are probably greatest in these former groupings. Thus it is from these types of innovation that any monopoly returns will be greatest, that contributions to overheads such as cost of capital, research and development and so on will be most abundant. This, of course, is precisely what Schumpeter's innovation theory would lead one to expect. The monopoly position provided by possessing a unique and important innovation shelters a firm from immediate competitive pressures and so enables it to charge a higher than competitive price.

On the other hand, a not insubstantial number of products in ranks 1 and 2 were priced at or relatively near to penetration levels. Why should firms behave in this way if they have a unique and valuable innovation to sell, and if they are also profit maximizers? The only explanation consistent with both the 'collusive/price insensitive hypothesis' and the simultaneous presence of successful high-priced innovations in these rankings is that of managerial misjudgement. (Although even this view would have to embrace the relaxing assumption that pharmaceutical firms follow a policy of price parallelism which is sufficiently flexible to allow for qualitative differences by innovation. Whether such flexibility could still be regarded as collusive behaviour is debatable.)

By contrast the 'effectively competitive' hypothesis would adopt the view that these products were subject to competitive pressures or had economic opportunities which the 'skimming priced' products were not or did not have. In an attempt to test this assertion Table 16.6 was constructed. This Table analyses all successful products in ranks 1 and 2 and indicates whether ('Yes') or not ('No') the innovation was superseded in periods t + 1 or t + 2.

Table 16.6

Analyses of successful products in therapeutic ranks 1 and 2, with or without succeeding innovations in periods t + 1 and t + 2

	Market success A		*Market success B*	
	Low price	*High price*	*Low price*	*High price*
Relative price I				
Yes	9	5	9	5
No	2	11	2	13
	Chi-squared: 4.8045		Chi-squared: 5.9675	
Relative price II				
Yes	7	4	8	6
No	6	10	5	10
	Chi-squared: 0.89		Chi-squared: 0.837	
Relative price III				
Yes	9	5	9	5
No	3	10	3	12
	Chi-squared: 3.1172		Chi-squared: 4.1713	
Relative price IV				
Yes	8	6	8	6
No	5	8	5	10
	Chi-squared: 0.343		Chi-squared: 0.637	

Yates's correction applied in all cases.

There is a visual indication in each of the subtables of Table 16.6 that products will tend to be introduced at a low rather than a high price if a superseding innovation (any value from 1 to 5) is expected. This would be completely in line with the theory of penetration and 'keep out' pricing. A low price policy would be adopted in anticipation of product competition in the near future as the original innovator attempted to carve out a suitably strong market position for himself. Such behaviour is also perfectly credible in the pharmaceutical industry where firms know each other's research and development (R and D) plans well in advance. (Clearly this is not the case with long-term R and D project selection plans, which will generally be highly confidential.) This advance knowledge will partly be due to scientific gossip, but more importantly will be due to the need to carry out the various formal tests for purposes of registration with the Medicines Commission. Clinical trials, in particular, are difficult to conceal from one's competitors. The statistical robustness of this economic inference is emphasized by the fact that, even for the small sample sizes under examination, the calculated chi-squared is close to or above the 5 per cent level of significance (3.841) in four of the eight cases, and this after application of the (in the circumstances) very rigorous Yates's correction.

III Conclusions

It seems, then, that firms adopt a whole range of pricing policies for innovations. The price charged for an innovation in relation to competitors is associated (in some more-or-less complex way) with the degree of therapeutic novelty that product has in relation to existing products. Prices are thus determined in large part by the level of competition perceived to exist in the market place. This depends in turn on the extent to which the innovation will provide a product (or characteristics) monopoly over existing product offerings. It is also dependent on whether such a monopoly is expected to be brief or prolonged. All of this is at odds with the thesis of those investigators who assert that there is no price competition in the industry, that prices are 'administered' and that doctors are price insensitive.

There is another interpretation, however. What we have not done is to provide evidence that prescribers are price sensitive. The data merely support the view that firms believe them to be so. It is difficult to credit, however, that full-time students of the pharmaceutical market (namely drug firm managers) are wrong, and that near to unanimously, in this belief. Further study of the data is required to identify definitively the causal relationship between price and market success. Moreover, the study has been restricted to the UK where it could be argued there is a strong monopsony buyer, the NHS, exerting countervailing power on the industry which has resulted in effectively competitive behaviour. A similar study to the one we have just reported, carried out in a country where such monopsony power does not exist would go a long way towards providing the necessary evidence to support or reject this latter hypothesis. Certainly this monopsony power appears to have brought about a lower overall price level in the UK than in many other countries (14). Casual theorizing, however, might lead one to reject the view that the monopsony cudgel, at least as epitomized by the VPRS, could produce the detailed, rational and competitive pricing behaviour which apparently exists. This for two main reasons. First, the study covered the prices of innovations in their first two or three years of life, from 1962 to 1970. The version of the VPRS which operated for every year (exclusive only of 1970) of this time span provided for either a two or a four year 'freedom period' during which firms could pitch prices at levels which they themselves considered appropriate. In short, the VPRS did not apply to innovations during most of the study period. Secondly, the 125 innovations were each compared with three or five existing products. That is, up to 750 different product prices were covered by this investigation. It seems improbable that the (unavoidably) limited scale, product-by-product negotiating style of the VPRS of the 1960s would produce the finely detailed results obtained here for such a large number of products.

Conversely, to the extent that the monopsonist is not dealing directly with firms (through the VPRS) but rather is operating through individual prescribers, each of whom has a certain amount of discretion, then the continual and formal attempts* by the Department of Health to encourage prescribers to be more price conscious may be at least partially responsible for the results we have obtained.

This leads to the interesting question as to whether in other countries with 'free' health care but with no ostensible exercise of monopsony power similar pricing patterns would be observed. One would, however, anticipate similar results in countries without a national health service; for example, the USA. There, doctors have long been aware that different patients have different incomes and so vary in ability to pay. This is reflected by their use of price discrimination and their levying of varying fees for the same treatment. It seems unlikely that such doctors will be price sensitive agents on behalf of their patients' needs for some parts of the total health care 'package' they provide but not for others (namely, drugs). If we bear in mind that the doctor will be assessing the cost effectiveness of a drug given the patient's total sociomedical needs it does seem probable that on occasion, if not many occasions, he will deliberately

*In particular, since 1968 all prescribers have received periodic circulars from the Department showing the comparative costs of different preparations available for treating similar diseases. Prior to this the main influence was mainly the indirect but wide publicity given by the national media to compulsory licensing litigation under either Sections 46 or 41 of the Patents Act. The cases in question generally revealed spectacular price differentials between the patented drug and the non-patented, generic chemical equivalent which the licensee applicant wished to market.

prescribe cheaper and/or older and/or less effective or less potent and/or generic, unbranded products. Also, there is the additional price constraint in the USA that the patient can shop around for the cheapest retail pharmacy to fill his prescription (resale price maintenance is illegal in many States). Patient price awareness of this sort will, *a priori,* also influence prescriber price consciousness. When the disease is one which requires continuous, repeat prescription therapy (e.g. rheumatism) as opposed to a single short period regimen (e.g. infections) this effect, *a fortiori,* will be enhanced.

What, if any, policy conclusions can be drawn from this discussion? Firms appear to behave in an 'effectively competitive' manner with regard to price. To the extent that doctors are price sensitive this is due either to the implications of their role as purchasing agents (in a private medical care system) or to the publicity given to price differentials (in a 'free' health care system). In the past, the VPRS may have had more impact on average price levels than on relative ones. *A priori,* this will be even more true for the 1970s now that the VPRS negotiations are explicitly linked to the firm's overall rate of return rather than primarily, as in the 1960s, to either comparative prices for the same drug in its main export markets, or alternatively to individual 'cost-plus' calculations. There is very little here to encourage sweeping allegations of monopolistic pricing behaviour in the pharmaceutical industry. However, until such time as evidence can be provided that doctors would be price sensitive in the absence of any patient/agency relationship, prudence would suggest we continue to assume that the low costs of providing British prescribers with intelligible comparative price information will yield substantial net benefits in terms of the industry's competitive performance.

References

1. Cooper, M.H. (1967). *Prices and Profits in the Pharmaceutical Industry,* p.43. Oxford, Pergamon.
2. Galbraith, J.K. (1967). *The New Industrial State,* p.110. Boston and New York, Houghton Mifflin; London, Andre Deutsch.
3. Comanor, W.S. (1964). Research and competitive product differentiation in the pharmaceutical industry in the United States. *Economica.* November, p.372.
4. Reekie, W. Duncan. (1975). *The Economics of the Pharmaceutical Industry,* p.37. London, Macmillan.
5. Monopolies Commission (1973). *Parallel Pricing.* Cmnd 5330. London, HMSO.
6. (1967). *Report of the Committee of Enquiry into the Relationship of the Pharmaceutical Industry with the National Health Service* (Sainsbury). Cmnd 3410, p.16.
7. Scherer, F.M. (1972). *Industrial Pricing,* pp.45-52. London and Chicago, Rand McNally.
8. Monopolies Commission (1973). *Chlordiazepoxide and Diazepam.* HC 197, paras. 218, 107, 244. London, HMSO.
9. Lall, Sanjaya (1974). The pharmaceutical industry and less developed countries, with special reference to India. *Bulletin of the Oxford Institute of Economics and Statistics.*

10. Dean, J. (1947). *Managerial Economics.* Englewood Cliffs, N.J., Prentice-Hall.
11. Reekie, W. Duncan. (1975). In: *Technical Appendix to the Canberra Hypothesis* Ed. by G. Teeling-Smith. Office of Health Economics.
12. Cooper, *Op.cit.*, p.244.
13. NEDO (1973). *Innovative Activity in the Pharmaceutical Industry.* National Economic Development Office.
14. Cooper, M.H. (1975). *European Pharmaceutical Prices, 1964-1974.* London, Croom Helm.

Part Four
Research

17

Priorities in Research

Sir Douglas Black

Any account of priorities must come to grips with a number of questions which seem simple and straightforward – at least until the time comes to answer them. These include the following:

What is a priority?
Whose priorities are they to be?
How are priorities to be arrived at?
What are the consequences of designating some area as a priority?

Before attempting to deal with these questions, I should make it clear that my present responsibility is for the general balance of the research programme of the Department from which I write, and not for specific research initiatives; it includes consideration of priorities for research, but not of priorities for service, which have recently been set out in a consultative document (1). While I have the natural interest in service priorities of any doctor who believes in the ideals of a National Health Service, I have no special information on them, nor responsibility for their development. While there should be some general concordance between priorities for research and priorities for service, there are special considerations which prevent them from being identical. In research, there are constraints of feasibility and scientific interest; in the services, constraints of facilities and manpower, which prevent a one-to-one relationship for their respective priorities. It should therefore be kept in mind that I have not studied the problems of priority definition for service to the same extent as I have studied those of priority definition for research. It is possible, however, that the approach based on 'indices of burden' which I shall describe, although developed in the research context, may also have relevance to service priorities, since it does not in itself involve the 'feasibility' constraints which enter at a later stage of the balance between 'service' and 'scientific' considerations.

What is a Priority?

The term 'priority' is sometimes used very loosely indeed, implying only what happens to be uppermost in the mind of an individual (or the consensus of a committee). In the context of research, a priority should perhaps be regarded as the outcome of a reasoned attempt to identify an area of activity which merits active steps, not merely to fund it, but to attract workers to it and to create a positive plan of action. This implies something more than the willingness to consider bids for support, which might be regarded as a rough and ready method of responding to what in effect are the priorities as seen by research workers themselves. It should perhaps be noted in passing that a *laissez-faire* attitude to the support of research, which relies implicitly on the good judgement of workers to propose research which is both 'interesting' and 'useful', has not in any rigorous way been discredited; it has not been shown to be inefficient on any objective criteria. But there are undeniably strong pressures towards the identification of socially based priorities for research, in partial distinction to the natural instinct of research workers to choose problems which offer a reasonable chance of solution. Such problems commonly arise in fields with which the research worker is already familiar, sometimes even identified. The contrary case is that it is for central authorities to study where research is most needed, and how it can then be fostered. On this view, it is not enough to leave judgements on research to the scientific community; they must be made aware of where the social pressures are greatest. The device chosen to achieve this end is twofold – a part of the funding of research has been transferred to Government Departments whose primary function is to maintain services; and within these Departments, the research managers are constrained to ensure that the research which they fund enjoys the support of 'customers', which in effect means those with administrative responsibility for services. Given that the ultimate decisions on research priorities will involve both social relevance and scientific feasibility, there is an element of tidiness in ascribing the 'relevance function' to the customers, and the 'feasibility function' to the contractors, i.e. the actual research workers. It is fairly obvious that a system of this kind will only work if there are confidence and understanding between customers and contractors; it is the task of research managers to bring this about. This immediately brings us to the second question in the list set out above.

Whose Priorities are They To Be?

It is not difficult to think of important advances which have been made by men who saw an objective clearly, and pursued it whole-heartedly. This consideration has been corporately expressed in the formation of 'pressure groups', dedicated to a concrete aim; and such groups have from time to time effectively stirred up the body politic. But the single-mindedness which gives such individuals and groups their strength also precludes them, in my view, from being good judges of general priorities. In pursuing the particular best, they may well be unwitting enemies of the general good. The fairest basis for priorities is no doubt the utilitarian one, the greatest benefit for the greatest number. The 'majority' implied in this statement is not perhaps 'silent'; but its voice tends to be confused, even discordant. Who is to be the judge, or at least the 'proxy customer'? There are three obvious possibilities – the Government and Parliament, broadly representing 'the people'; the Health Departments and National Health Service, representing predominantly service interests; and the Research Councils, representing the research community. Each of these has strengths and weaknesses. The Government and Parliament are democratically elected, and are most directly susceptible to 'the consumer interest', and least influenced by professional pressures; but they certainly have other things to do, and the most notable example of government priority-making in the medical research field, the Nixon assault on cancer, has not been very encouraging in its results to date. The Health Departments have the strength of responsible contact with the health problems of the nation, and have access to in-house statistical and economic advice, and to the Office of Population Censuses and Surveys; they are, however, and quite rightly, preoccupied with service matters, and, in relation to bio-medical research at least, they are not well placed to assess the feasibility, as opposed to the desirability, of research proposals. The Research Councils are dedicated to maintaining the research capacity of the nation, and in pursuance of this aim they have over the years developed close links with the academic community, from whom indeed their independent members are largely recruited; and they have developed effective techniques for the management and the assessment of research. The Medical Research Council has a lay Chairman and a number of lay members, but the membership is predominantly 'scientific'. In my own view, this is justified by the nature of the issues with which they mainly have to deal; but as a professional myself, I might not carry full conviction with those hostile critics who see the Council as a defender of the research community, rather than as a servant of the public acting through Government. My own view, perhaps something of a compromise, is that each of these three agencies has an important role. Because of the manifold other preoccupations of Government, the main dialogue must be between the Health Departments, with a bias towards social needs, and the Research Councils, with a bias towards feasibility and other scientific considerations. But the Government and Parliament have the ultimate responsibility of ensuring that the system is serving the broad public interests of health and medical science. As an aid to the exercise of this responsibility, both the Health Departments and the Research Councils make annual reports to Parliament.

How are Priorities to be Arrived At?

First of all, not by a monopoly system. It is entirely good that much medical research is funded by voluntary organizations and by industry, and that much of the publicly funded medical research takes place in the universities, independently of centrally promulgated priorities. Rothschild's (2) stigmatization of chance observations as 'a form of scientific roulette' does not seem to me to dispose of their value; after all, there have been some winners in that particular game, and many skilled players who might not have benefited from central advice.

It is good that scientific *laissez-faire* – which really means the judgements of responsible independent scientists – should be conserved in the important sectors mentioned above. This in no way relieves us of the obligation of defining priorities in the massive sector of medical research which is funded directly, as such, by Government through the Health Departments and the Medical Research Council. For many years past, the Council has defined and published the areas to which it attaches priority; and the Health Departments have had an input to this process through the attendance of their Chief Medical Officers at the Clinical Research Board. Following the 1972 White Paper on Government Research and Development (3), the input of the Health Departments to the Medical Research Council has been formalized and strengthened in various ways. There are four nominees of Government Departments on the Council itself (two from the Department of Health and Social Security, one from the Scottish Home and Health Department and one from the Department of Employment). There are three Departmental nominees on each of the Council's main Boards, whose meetings are also attended by a Departmental Board Liaison Officer, and by the Chief Scientists of the DHSS and SHHD. Departmental officers from the Research Management Division take part in detailed activities of the Council, such as Conferences, Working Parties, and visits to research establishments. These officers maintain contact with the divisions of the Department which have responsibility for service, and can thus transmit detailed views on priorities as seen in the Health Departments. These 'priorities of detail' are arrived at within the service divisions, assisted by specialist advisers.

The definition of the major priorities for biomedical research is a difficult process, in which social considerations and considerations of feasibility and likelihood of practical results all enter. On the face of it, the primary responsibility for defining social needs might seem to lie with the Health Departments, and for defining the scientific realities with the Council. But this is an over-simplification, since the Department have access to expert biomedical advice through the Chief Medical Officer's advisory system; and the Council have throughout their history taken social needs into full account. Neither social needs nor scientific feasibility are readily quantifiable, since in various ways they both involve value judgements. We still have much to learn about the ways in which priorities can be arrived at, but I can give an account of the present state of partnership between the Departments and the Council.

In a statement to the Subcommittee on Health of the US Senate Committee on Labor and Public Welfare, Kerr White asked, and to a large extent answered, the key question:

'On whose list of health problems are the behavioral and biomedical scientists of the country to work? Who draws up the list, and on what is it to be based – the perceived needs of the public, the curiosity of the investigators, or a sensible balance between the two? We require personal compassion for the care of individual patients, but statistical compassion for establishing public policy.'

Role of the Health Departments. That striking phrase, 'the perceived needs of the public' conceals two important questions – 'Who are "the public"?', and 'Who is to do the perceiving?'. Furthermore, how are the perceptions to be translated into manageable proposals for research? This is the difficult task which faces a Department, anxious to produce a meaningful input, based on social needs. The obvious solution, of carrying out attitude surveys to find out the public's own perception of its needs, seems to me to lack practicality. Healthy people have a healthy disinterest in illness, which constitutes one of the main barriers to the preventive approach – a barrier which must be overcome by advances in the behavioural sciences, if we are to make radical improvements in the nation's health. As an alternative, in the desperate search for something tangible, my colleague David Pole and I have begun to explore an approach based on indices of the burden imposed by various diseases on the health services, and on people. Our first analysis has been published (4), and I shall only outline the approach here. We used 52 broad categories of disease, and determined for each one of them the share of five 'indices of burden' for which it was responsible. Two of the indices were related to hospitals – days of bed occupancy, and out-patient attendances. Our index for primary care included both surgery attendances and home visits. The fourth index, which applies only to the insured population, was days of Sickness Benefit. The fifth index was 'loss of life expectancy', based on mortality statistics. Partly no doubt because of the breadth of the disease categories used, the number of conditions which together accounted for 50 per cent of the burden on any single index was small, ranging from 3 to 9. There was, however, considerable disparity between the indices as regards the predominant conditions. For example, while mental diseases and mental handicap are major causes of hospitalization and sickness absence, they contribute little to mortality. Tumours and arterial diseases are major causes of mortality and of hospitalization, but come far behind respiratory diseases as causes of sickness-absence. For our first analysis, we took a straight average of the five indices, which gives the list in Table 17.1, which at least indicates that only 11 categories out of 52 account for 70 per cent of the total burden.

Table 17.1

Category	*Percentage of total burden*
Mental illness and handicap	14
Respiratory disease	13
Ischaemic heart disease	7
Bone and joint disease	6
Accident and Suicide	6
Neoplasms	6
Digestive disorders	5
Neurological disorders	4
Cerebrovascular disease	4
Skin disease	3
Urogenital disease	2
All Others	30

By concentrating on indices for which figures are available, this analysis leaves out what has been called the 'misery factor'. Much suffering, some of it remediable, may not be brought to medical attention, or may call on it only infrequently. Another cause of under-representation of particular conditions lies in the quirks of taxonomy. To give a specific example, skin disorders are certainly underestimated in importance, both because they cause prolonged misery, without usually leading to hospitalization or home visits; and skin infections and tumours are indexed under 'infections' and 'tumours', and not under 'skin disease'. The extent of this underestimation can be gauged by comparing our figure of 4.84 per cent of the primary care load attributable to skin disorders with other surveys, presumably including infections and tumours, which give figures around 10 per cent.

The assumption that the burdens represented by these indices are of equal importance is decidedly weak, though we felt compelled to make it as the only alternative to value judgements for which we had no established basis. There are two obvious ways in which the approach could be developed. The indices used could be weighted in terms of the relative cost of the burden imposed – easy in the case of Sickness Benefit; difficult in the case of in-patient beds, because of the range of costs between different types of hospital; more difficult still in evaluating 'loss of life expectancy'. This approach is equally vulnerable to the criticism that it omits the 'misery factor'; but in view of the escalating costs of certain services, it may still be worth making. An alternative would be to recognize that each burden implies an objective – to save beds, to lessen attendances at out-patient clinics and, in primary care, to diminish illness in the working population, or to prevent premature death. If any politician or publicist were brave enough to rank these prior objectives in order of importance, the corresponding indices could be weighted accordingly.

Role of the Medical Research Council. To quote from the Council's 1974-75 Annual Report, 'Biomedical research is concerned with improving the future well-being of the community and of its individual members. All the research supported by the Council is directed at that objective and, in order to ensure its continuing attainment, the Council is also concerned with the support and maintenance of the country's scientific capability in its medical disciplines.' The Council thus has the task of giving practical expression to priorities, whether these are communicated to them by the Health Departments or generated by discussion within the Council or its Boards. Detailed scientific issues of feasibility and merit are usually first discussed within the Boards, on the basis of submissions made by subgroups expert in particular fields; at this stage, a Health Department input of objectives, as seen by them, is introduced. The submissions of the Boards are consolidated by Council, and become the basis of a 'Forward Look' submission, made to the Advisory Board for the Research Councils, which has the responsibility of allocating the Science Vote among the five Research Councils. One factor in decisions on allocation is the extent to which Councils can be seen to have considered and made explicit their perception of national needs.

When it comes to translating these into actual research, priorities become very detailed, and for such details I would refer the reader to successive Annual Reports of the Council, which describe in detail the development of the Council's scientific policy. About one-quarter of the Council's research is now funded on a commission basis from the Health Departments, and recent reports give some information on commissioned research.

What are the Consequences of Designating an Area as a Priority?

There would be little point in a search for priorities, if no action were to follow their definition. However, the action required varies with the nature of the problem to which the statement of priority directs attention. This is clearly recognized by the effective agents for biomedical research, the Council, who distinguish three categories of priority in respect of the action to be taken. Some health problems are of such manifest importance that, even though no new initiatives are immediately apparent, there must be continued alertness to support proposals for research within these areas. The areas currently designated in this category are arterial disease and mental health (which correspond closely to what might be derived from the indices of burden); microbial disease, which by its pervasiveness escapes the taxonomic net of the burden approach; and environmental factors in diseases, which have great importance to the Department of Employment, as well as to the Health Departments.

The second category of priorities relates to areas where there are obvious opportunities for expanding the research effort, and where the problem and possible initiatives to solve it have been made the subject of a special study. The category includes both problems such as cancer, which comes high on the burden approach, and deafness, which is not high on the burden approach, but are the cause of great misery and public concern.

The third category of priorities relates to the responsibility of the Council for 'the support and maintenance of the country's scientific capability'. These priorities relate to disciplines in which there is a recognized shortage of trained investigators. For example, there are absolute shortages of trained research workers in epidemiology and psychiatry; while in clinical neurology and dentistry, the service burdens are so great as to leave little time for practitioners to engage in original work.

In the present state of resource restriction, compounded by residual inflation, there is little prospect of poor work being supported in any area, even were that desirable; and new initiatives have to be matched by retrenchment in other areas. Nevertheless, money does become available from the cessation of short-term projects, and even, on a longer timescale, of programmes of research. Worthwhile research on difficult problems does, however, require sustained effort; and the investment of the Council in its own units and establishments is really the only way in which it can produce sustained effort, and at the same time maintain in being a research resource on which it can call directly. Aside from the falling-in of projects, another area of flexibility lies in the Council's training awards, whose distribution among disciplines is reviewed annually, providing the opportunity to encourage recruitment to particular research disciplines. The Council can also support new and important disciplines by setting up units in universities, selected after tenders invited from them. For example, clinical genetics was largely fostered by the Council in the 1950s and has now taken root in the medical schools. More recently, similar initiatives have been taken in clinical pharmacology and in reproductive biology. The full value of initiatives of this kind does, however, depend in the long term on the ability of the universities to disseminate such disciplines throughout the medical schools, a task which is beyond the Council's own resources.

Conclusion

Limitation of space has led me to focus this account on priorities in biomedical research. Similar principles, and similar practical limitations, no doubt apply in other areas. The essence of the priority problem seems to me to lie in how to achieve clarity on the prior objectives for research, and then to relate these both to the social burden imposed by the various problems and to the likelihood of their solution. There are considerable uncertainties in both of these assessments, so there must always be a place for the chartered libertines of research, whose motivation is instructed curiosity.

References

1. Department of Health and Social Security (1976). *Priorities for Health and Personal Social Services in England.* London, HMSO.
2. Rothschild, Lord (Chairman) (1972). *The Organisation and Management of Government R & D. in a Framework for Government Research and Development.* Cmnd 4814. London, HMSO.
3. White Paper (1972). *Government Research and Development.* Cmnd 5046. London, HMSO.
4. Black, D.A.K. and Pole, J.D. (1975). Priorities in biomedical research: indices of burden. *British Journal of Preventive and Social Medicine,* 29, 222.

18

Priorities in Laboratory Research

L. Mary Pickford

This chapter will concern itself with laboratory research. It is written by one who has been interested in basic biological research but whose aim has always been that, in the long run, the results should be of use to man. Inevitably there will be bias and selection. Perhaps this is to the good as it will stimulate argument.

Epidemiology, as against laboratory research, is complementary to the latter because it shows, amongst other things, the kinds of diseases which are prevalent, where they occur geographically and how far, if at all, they are related to race and habit of life. Social research is also important because no man is truly healthy who lacks a reasonable degree of contentment. Humans are infinitely varied in their needs, sensitivities and likes so that it is highly desirable that all regulations and plans should be as flexible as possible, and that man should never be used as a mere robot in a striving for efficiency. This applies to laboratory workers as well as the general populace. From the outset it must be made clear that the writer abhors the idea that there should be a central and/or governmental control of research programmes, believing that the outcome would be disastrous. Almost inevitably, those in control would become more and more office-ridden and remote from what is possible and profitable. Scientific initiative and morale would be sapped. The great majority of scientists, medical and otherwise, have a sense of responsibility and do not try merely to satisfy their own curiosity. The system of autonomous research councils such as the Medical Research Council and the Agricultural Research Council works admirably and has enabled British scientists to be productive in both quality and quantity. The system is envied by less fortunate countries.

Happily for medicine, because the effects of disease fall into fairly clear patterns, the variations are of a relatively minor character and it is possible to describe 'typical' cases and to provide guide-lines for their treatment. The extreme exceptions are few but interesting. However, we know little about the causes of individual differences, how far they are truly somatic and how far they are emotional. It follows that emotion must be defined; in some it may have a biochemical component, in others this may be combined with conditioning and environment. On this subject there are more hypotheses than facts and information is urgently needed, since mental imbalance and illness abound. Neurological disorders also are many.

Money is needed for laboratory research, and when money is in short supply it is urgently necessary to try to group research programmes in order of relative importance. In one system of grouping, programmes that seem to be approaching an end-point or milestone may be placed first, regardless of whether the results will benefit few or many; second will be those problems in which the work will not mature for some years; and third, work determining basic facts not aimed at immediate practical benefit. This grouping is founded on hope and possibilities rather than probabilities. It will be recalled that great expectations arose for the treatment of rheumatoid arthritis when cortisone first became available. It was thought that at last there was a breakthrough. Numerous investigations were encouraged but the high hopes were not fulfilled. However, the work was not wasted as it aided other, and apparently unrelated, subjects.

Another method of grouping laboratory research is to relate it to current needs of the population; that is, it is 'consumer' orientated. Again this is an exercise in speculation. One has only to consider the enormous amount of time and money spent on cancer research and the incommensurate results. Certainly advances have been made, but not in proportion to the amount of energy expended. But again the work has not been wasted as much of it can be applied in other fields. In the present time of financial stringency it has been recommended that this second method should be used and resources go towards attempts to unravel a limited number of current problems in the hope that this will lead to the greatest good for the greatest number. Where a problem is a straightforward technical one, results may well appear in a short time. Our technical knowledge is far in advance of our biological understanding and, it may be added, our general wisdom. One trouble with 'consumer' orientated research is that, by the time the research is well under way, for reasons we do not always understand, the disease in question becomes less common and another takes its place. Another difficulty is that research is an exploration of the unknown; the prospect may seem good and the preliminary study well done but, owing to our ignorance, we do not know where we shall arrive nor how long it will take to get there. Nevertheless, some useful information should accrue on the way, however much it may differ from that anticipated. Ideally, every *good* research worker deserves support.

The diseases that loom large in the Western world are those of the brain and peripheral nervous system, the circulation, and the joints and muscles.

Many other disorders affect a smaller number of people and may give rise to just as much misery. If any advance is to be made in understanding the causes and prevention of disease, basic (i.e. laboratory) sciences must receive their share of help. Pathology can tell us what has happened, physiology and biochemistry can try to tell us how the organism ought to work and where it may have gone astray, and pharmacology can do far more than provide drugs for treatment. The need for bacteriology is obvious. Perhaps the most complex and inaccessible organ is the central nervous system and it is here that the basic sciences can certainly be of use. Slowly we are discovering the many transmitters in the central nervous system, their sites of action and the pathways affected by them. The pharmacologists can help by developing antagonists and blocking agents for the transmitters. These, used together with stereotaxic recording, stimulation and destruction of accurately localized areas may and have given us the positive and negative pictures showing the path taken by external and internal stimuli and the influence of these on bodily behaviour and function. Then in due time, perhaps a long time, it may be possible to produce drugs even more specific than any existing ones, for the control of chosen neuronal activities. This would obviate the controversial and irreversible use of surgery in cases such as excessive aggression.

Where mental disease is concerned we need to know the age group chiefly involved. This information must already be available. We must expect the problems of age to remain with us for the simple reason that the expectation of life is greater than it was. Whether we shall be able to limit the amount of senility and degeneration depends upon an increased knowledge of the process of ageing. Observation shows that the ageing process is not necessarily accompanied by mental and bodily helplessness. We do not know how far this depends on heredity and how far on habits of life. At the present time there is pressure to maintain a degree of youthfulness in women after the menopause by the administration of oestrogens. It appears that some women certainly benefit. Apart from the question of safety, we do not know whether aged tissues react like young ones to the hormone, nor whether it is not oestrogens alone that are needed. Possibly a mixture of hormones is required. In the younger age groups depression, schizophrenia and breakdown from stress predominate. We have little knowledge of the causes and pathology of schizophrenia and not a great deal about the other two. But in all three instances there are drugs that can aid recovery. All these mental conditions are a serious strain on the economy either directly or indirectly. Maintaining the incapacitated is expensive because a healthy productive individual has to spend time caring for them. Without a true vocation this occupation can lead to mental imbalance.

Cardiovascular disorders often kill (coronary block) or seriously disable (stroke) at a time of life when the individual should still be useful and may have a growing family to support. Again the result is expense and unhappiness. Much work has already been done and facts accumulated, but except in a few instances (smoking, too little exercise and too much food) it is not wholly clear what is cause and what effect. Until later life, males and females tend to have different types of cardiovascular disease, which suggests that the pattern may be related to the concentration and proportion of circulating sex hormones. Perhaps it would be possible in some way to counteract the harmful effect of the hormones without disturbing their normal action on the reproductive organs and libido. If this could be done, it might lead to a reduction in mental disorders of vascular origin. Another obscure sex-related observation is that before the fifth decade more females than males are affected by myasthenia gravis.

Here alone is a huge field demanding investigation and to that may be added joint and muscle diseases, both of them crippling and distressing. Other disorders may not afflict such large numbers of people, but that does not mean that they are unimportant and may be neglected. It is satisfactory to see that efforts are being made by the Medical Research Council to encourage research in dermatology. Certain skin conditions, such as severe psoriasis, can be an almost unbearable handicap; others are treated as minor matters and of little real importance. This is not always true. A condition not visible to the public eye may be irritating in more senses than one and lead to bad temper, impatience and difficulties for family and working life. A visible disorder, particularly in the young, can lead to permanent mental instability.

There are a large number of temporarily disabling illnesses, in particular respiratory and digestive. Some of these are self-induced by smoking and unwise eating, others are acquired accidentally from infection and lack of hygiene. But there remain a number that are not so easily explained away, such as asthma and gastric and duodenal ulcers. Here we return to a basic science and the problem of immunity to foreign substances and autoimmunity. As a result of work on the former, many infections can be prevented or rendered mild. And for some years now it has become clear that autoimmunity is a factor in many diseases. More work is needed.

Another and highly controversial subject demands mention; namely, the prenatal diagnosis of fetal abnormalities, especially in older women and those with a history of bearing abnormal infants. The woman can be tested and, if thought necessary, offered abortion. To those who believe this unethical and wholly unnecessary it can only be said that others sincerely believe it proper for the happiness of parents, and the abnormal child and siblings, not to mention the State. The parents do not have to accept abortion and the mother learns the possibility of an abnormal infant before the mentally critical postpartum period. Nowadays abnormal children may well survive their parents and have to be handed over to the care of strangers. This means life-long anxiety for the parents and ultimate distress for the children. There are already good tests, via amniocentesis, for Down's syndrome, anencephaly and spina bifida. Better ones are needed that give speedy answers and are, as nearly as possible, 100 per cent accurate. The essence of the matter is that, if abortion is to be performed, it must be done as early as possible and it must never prove to have been unnecessary. At present, should amniocentesis suggest abnormality, other and more expensive tests may be used for confirmation. Also coming under the heading of controversial subjects is that of contraceptives. Much work is being done on these, not only for women but for men also. More needs to be done in a search for reversible methods and because of the occasional side-effects of the existing ones. Here we return to the problem of individual variation. When oral contraceptives are used, why is it that some women successfully adapt to the raised concentration of circulating angiotensin when others do not? And again, why do some women suffer thrombotic episodes? Both groups of women appear to be equally 'healthy'.

Epidemiology and social research help to show that certain problems need special encouragement. This does not mean that the given subjects must of necessity take precedence over others, nor that practical results will follow research. It has already been pointed out as self-evident that we cannot foresee the answer to the unknown. The future value of work must be judged not only by the subject and the plan of work but also and importantly by the quality and experience of the worker. If he/she is a senior then the record of achievement is available for inspection. If he/she is young or a beginner, then the laboratory in which the work is to be done is an invaluable pointer to quality or otherwise. Admittedly, choosing quality throws responsibility on the departmental chief supporting the application and on the body financing the project. But it can and has been done successfully. Probably outstanding medical difficulties will attract a large number of workers; therefore there will be little need to advertise major problems, only those that have received less attention.

The following is the writer's choice of the subjects that urgently demand more basic knowledge: cardiovascular system, central and peripheral nervous systems, joints and muscles and skin. Under the heading of cardiovascular system is included the problem of deep vein thrombosis. Tests for fetal abnormalities in selected cases have been mentioned; also simple and reversible contraception. Where the latter is concerned it must be remembered that the world is populated by people of unequal intelligence and opportunity; a system of contraception suited to one group is not necessarily suited to another whose need is as great. The manner in which these problems can be approached is infinitely varied and all the basic sciences are concerned. A point to be made is that drugs can be used as tools as well as for treatment. The same is true of immune reactions. The latter are proving their value in the assay of minute amounts of certain substances present in body fluids. Also needed are techniques for blocking or reversing autoimmunity and neoplastic growth. Individual and sex variations in the response to events, diseases and drugs are interesting and important. Exceptions may give a clue to normal processes. Some questions may be posed that demonstrate our ignorance. Why does multiple sclerosis predominantly attack the central nervous system in some people and in others the peripheral nerves? Why does myasthenia gravis occasionally affect mainly the ocular muscles and the myasthenic syndrome those of the shoulder and pelvic girdles? How far are the minute and gross anatomy of the individual responsible for the differences, or do these depend on the nature of the toxins and immune processes? Clearly, little basic experimental work can be done on man, though ultimately it is applied to him. Work on isolated animal cells and tissues should not be decried. It can suggest what to look for in the whole animal. This paragraph adds up to the fact that basic research in any subject is worth doing. However, some subjects are more likely than others to produce useful results in a relatively short time; which these are is a matter of luck as much as judgement. This statement is not as nihilistic as it may seem, but for those who do not work in the clinical field or in a biological laboratory it cannot be stressed too strongly that research is rather like prayer. The answer is unpredictable. Properly used, the answer will prove useful sometime, somewhere. Finally, an occasional criticism made of research that is that too much of it is repetitive and therefore wasteful. There is a small fragment of truth in this. Nowadays the literature is so vast that it is sometimes difficult to know what is being done. Also, from the references given, it *appears* that only a few writers pay attention to experiments done more than 20-25 years ago. Research in the past was performed with relatively simple equipment and methods but a striking fact about much of it is the excellence and accuracy of the observations. A great deal of this older work deserves to be remembered and might well save time now.

The economics of research depend upon a number of factors. If the worker holds a university or other salaried post, then his requirement will be for expenses only. On occasion an assistant will be needed. Where maintenance is required, at the present time and at the bottom of the scale, it will approximate to £3,000 per annum and for a technician about £2,000 or more depending on his experience. Expenses for materials vary with the problem and may be £500-£1,000 per annum. Many laboratories already have a supply of sophisticated equipment which can almost certainly be shared by several workers, but where equipment is lacking, present costs are high. Analysis of biological material that is tagged with a radioactive substance is rapid and accurate, which means that a large number of results can be obtained in a short time. Geiger counters cost from £7,000 to £10,000. Autoanalysers may cost as much as £60,000 and can run through a number of selected analyses with great speed, needing only very small quantities of material. Spectrophotometers and oscilloscopes cost about £5,000-10,000; six-channel recorders about £6,000. Computers suitable for laboratory work cost up to £10,000, depending on their complexity. Gas chromatographs are, again, very expensive; from £3,000 upwards. The advantages of these items is their accuracy and speed in analysis, calculation and consideration of the effect of variables that may influence the results of experimental techniques. One of their disadvantages is that a fault developing suddenly at a critical moment is not easily corrected and may mean the loss of days or months of work and expensive materials. They also demand the availability of an expert technician who can deal with minor faults; that is, another salaried worker must be employed. On the whole, modern electronic and other machines do not fail often; but, where possible, it is as well to have as a stand-by a robust old-fashioned recording or other device. For many purposes they are still useful and adequate.

Of late there has been much discussion about the price of drugs. There is a review available of the work and costs necessary for the production of even one therapeutically useful drug. The cost may be from £7 to 10 million and the time 5-10 years before devising, testing and licensing are completed. Only after that can profits begin to be made for ploughing back into further work. In the course of the work it is possible that other substances of experimental interest will be made.

In summary, then, if there is a technical problem, it is likely that it can be solved fairly quickly. If the problem is biological there can be no guarantee that the results of a given line of research will solve it quickly or tidily. Encouragement may hopefully be given to those working in certain selected fields. The chances are that something useful will appear, though it may be unexpected and unrelated to the original problem and further time must pass before it can be applied to a practical purpose. Nowadays costs are high, but modern equipment enables the performance of experiments not otherwise possible and can give rapid and accurate results. However, for those unable to obtain large grants, it should not be forgotten that with ingenuity there are still many useful and relatively simple observations and analyses that can be made by those determined to work.

Bibliography

Buchanan, W. Watson and Dick, W. Carson (Eds.) (1976) *Recent Advances in Rheumatology*, Parts I & II. Edinburgh and London, Churchill Livingstone.

Hagard, S. and Carter, F.A. (1976). Preventing the birth of infants with Down's syndrome: a cost-benefit analysis. *British Medical Journal*, **1**, 753-756.

Maddox, J. (1975). *Pharmaceutical Research and Public Ownership*. Published by the Association of British Pharmaceutical Industries.

Prevention of Coronary Heart Disease. (1976). A Report of the Joint Working Party of the Royal College of Physicians of London and the British Cardiac Society.

Rothschild, Lord (Chairman) (1971). *The Organisation and Management of Government Research and Development*. Cmnd 4814. London, HMSO.

Epilogue

Calbert I. Phillips and J.N. Wolfe

Are there possibilities for achieving greater economic realism in Medicine? We have selected some points made by our contributors for comment, but each chapter must be read in full to counteract our bias.

The *individual* may have enough common sense to accept less than perfect physical and mental well-being, and to differentiate between trivial symptoms susceptible to self-medication and potentially serious complaints (Wade and Kendell). Fry mentions some observations made in a group of 12 general practices over a 10-year period; there was a fall of 60% in home visits and 16% in office consultations. His own performance over a 25-year period was a reduction of 90% and 33% respectively. This is attributed to his greater experience, better organization, delegation to paramedical personnel and more patient involvement in their own treatment. This change has not been accompanied by an increase in referrals to specialists: over the 25-year period, these have fallen by half. On the other hand, the knowledge that a comprehensive medical service is readily available – Woodruff's 'fire brigade' principle – may relieve the individual of a major source of anxiety throughout his life. However, insurance (of which this is a variant) is expensive, and the optimal amount required is generally less than the maximum amount possible.

The school health service, the value of which needs critical assessment (McCrae), might usefully teach children hygiene, dietetics, the value of exercise, the prevention of accidents and the dangers of smoking, alcohol and other drugs. Prevention allows a healthy individual to remain so, whereas treatment often can only make a sick person less sick. It is surprising that more 'advanced' countries which have achieved so much in public health have done so little for individually based prevention of diseases associated with abundance of resources.

Decision making, especially diagnosis, is so central to the problem of Medicine that we have included five chapters dealing with different aspects of it. Even if economy in logical processes were not psychologically and aesthetically attractive, these writers would be unanimous in arguing that discrimination in the collection of evidence, and economy in the construction and refutation of hypotheses can achieve financial savings. Campbell condemns the 'mindless work-up' and Dudley, using the principle of Bayes's theorem, advocates the *sequential* collection of the limited basis required for a confident diagnosis. Similar considerations apply to decisions about whether any treatment is required and the choice of treatment.

The mind recognizes patterns easily. Diagnostic inference seems likely to be analogous to pattern recognition and both seem to utilize dependent probabilities. However, dependent probabilities are difficult to estimate from small samples. To put one aspect of that differently, an *experienced* doctor will make a diagnosis or a decision with less irrelevant information than the inexperienced (Campbell and Dudley). Some of the waste, inefficiency and duplication in the National Health Service is attributable to its dependence on inexperienced junior doctors. These are greater in number than are required to fill the anticipated permanent vacancies; Brocklehurst favours more direct involvement of the consultant in patient care. An implication is that the savings in salaries of the junior staff and the savings in their expensive clinical habits (Campbell) would go far towards paying for any increase in establishment of consultants required. Of course there is a trade-off between the wisdom of experience and the enthusiasm and modern training of the young.

Some of the recent increase in medical staffing has been due to greater leisure expectations of medical graduates compared with the hours of work tolerated by the single-handed, single-minded entrepreneur of 40 years ago. These considerations suggest a reassessment of the increasing numbers being produced by our medical schools as well as a reconsideration of the basic principles of their clinical training.

In any organization with an end-product which is difficult to measure, staffing should be inadequate, as a matter of policy. In Medicine, a clinician will still have the freedom to decide his own priorities. This is an application of Parkinson's law: 'Work expands so as to fill the time available for its completion', which can be expressed more concisely as 'The devil finds work for idle hands to do'.

Voluntary individual private audit. Peer group influence is probably better than central control, but is expensive in time and effort and cannot in practice extend into every activity of the doctor, from the trivial (which, summed, can be expensive) to the major. A voluntary individual private audit applied at every stage in patient management could effect major savings. The motivated expert is the best person to discriminate between value and cost. A professional person should act responsibly to the community as well as to his patient. Likewise the patient also must act sensibly, but if an individual believes that the community does not place enough value on his life, his health or his time, we assume the individual's right to divert his own personal resources to pay for private medical care. The possibilities for economies mentioned in this volume would apply as cogently for the individual or an insurance company as for a state-financed or state-subsidized system of health care.

Automation and computer-assisted systems are the usual method for escaping from the constraints of a labour-intensive industry. Whitby shows how they have produced a disproportionate increase in output from laboratories of clinical chemistry with a limited increase in staff. This is to some extent an exception to the Rule of Parsimony in Medicine. He does, however, mention a recent investigation which has shown that an extravagance of information produced by 'admission-screening' makes no difference to the outcome for the patient. The problem of the contamination of a multiplicity of tests by an occasional false-positive is well known. It may be an over-simplification to suggest that a chance has been missed to centralize laboratories more, in spite of the problems of transport and communication.

Some outstanding discoveries can be immediately accepted as valid on *a priori* grounds or after minimal trial. Many, however, require validation by randomized clinical trials as described and discussed by Ederer. Since the use of a randomized clinical trial implies doubt about the results, strict adherence to its principles, especially true randomization of controls and avoidance of the possibility of observer bias, is essential, especially when new treatments are likely to be applied on a world-wide scale. Ederer mentions examples of erroneous conclusions when the rules are infringed. The importance of the randomized clinical trial is emphasized in other papers, especially that by Kerr and Parboosingh, and also those by McCrae and Jennett. Statistics should receive more attention in the undergraduate medical curriculum, not because many students will do research, but because they will acquire criteria by which to assess critically innovations for which unjustified claims are made. More stringent statistical standards by medical journals for accepting articles for publication would encourage investigators towards better planning and execution of their researches, and more cautious interpretation of their results. Even if statistical significance has been demonstrated in research of high quality, economic significance has to be considered if the benefit is slight and the cost high.

Around 10% of the cost of the NHS is absorbed by the pharmaceutical services. 'Is any drug necessary?' is a question which should precede 'What drug should be prescribed?'. Another important question is 'What is the exact amount required for the course of treatment?' Even in a wide variety of established mental diseases in patients in a mental hospital, Rollin provides good evidence – though not based on a strict randomized clinical trial – that withdrawal of all treatment produced improvement in many, while in a few there remained some residual symptoms controlled on a smaller or intermittent dose. That must apply often in trivial and self-limiting complaints. Wade shows that fashion and individual, regional and national preferences or prejudices affect the amount and type of drugs prescribed. Although Reekie's statistics provide evidence that the pharmaceutical industry is price-sensitive, and presumably the doctors are also, there may be considerable scope for economy in prescribing. Expensive drugs should not be given for inappropriate illnesses. The cheapest, simplest drug available should be prescribed if it is equally effective. Surgeons are also susceptible to fashion in their choice of operation (see Ederer's list).

The obstetricians and paediatricians say that improvement in standard of living may well explain much of the reduction in maternal, perinatal and infant mortality and morbidity over the years, although improved medical care may claim a proportion of the credit. The obstetricians suggest that a critical appraisal is required of the current trends towards a specialist hospital-centred service while a community-based service using general practitioners and midwives may be more appropriate. The current activism in obstetric practice, which is expensive, clearly requires a randomized clinical trial or multivariate analysis, at least to assess the value of induction of labour and continuous fetal monitoring in labour. It is unfortunate that epidural anaesthesia is extremely expensive, requiring 24-hour specialist cover.

While conservation of scarce resources should be applied in the situation wherein a patient consults a doctor, altogether more stringent standards of cost benefit and other properties must be considered when the community offers to individuals immunization or screening for the early detection of disease. Some screening and immunization programmes have been very successful, e.g. for phenylketonuria and poliomyelitis respectively, but in many the benefit is doubtful (amniocentesis and chromosome analysis in mothers aged less than, say, 40 years) or even poor (cystic fibrosis). In such cases the dilemma between the individual's interests and society's responsibility can be acute. 'The public' is probably not very concerned about the absence of a service for diagnosis of Down's syndrome (mongolism) in early pregnancy for the few women over 40 who would know in time and accept termination, and even less concerned to provide universal immunization, for example against whooping cough. These attitudes probably arise from an implicit public distinction between 'Acts of God', like Down's syndrome, and 'Acts of Man', like the unfortunate occasional serious complication of immunization. Some rationalization of this attitude may be developed in terms of a distinction between mean outcome – which appeals to epidemiologists – and a range or variance of outcome which attracts disproportionate attention, understandably enough, by dramatic individual examples.

The poor quality of life for many babies who have survived severe spina bifida as a result of operations and antibiotic treatment has made paediatricians and neurosurgeons more selective in their choice of babies for treatment. Analysis of the pregnant mother's blood for alpha-feto protein has a moderately high probability of revealing the presence of fetuses with 'open' spina bifida, etc., which may well reduce the numbers of affected children being born.

As mortality decreases, the effect of morbidity on the quality of life requires more consideration. The concept of *utilities* of states of health has been introduced, but their quantitative estimation raises serious problems (Card).

The neurosurgeon has difficulty in assessment of cases of brain damage from injury and other diseases, especially in the hitherto economically productive. Between cure and care, a category 'rescue' is becoming more important (Jennett). Artificial means for maintaining life have made more obvious the need to diagnose 'brain death' which is generally accepted as allowing withdrawal of life-support measures, or avoidance of their use. This is a re-statement in a modern context of the long-established principle in Medicine (from *The Latest Decalogue* by Arthur Hugh Clough):

'Thou shalt not kill, but need'st not strive
Officiously to keep alive'

It also applies in geriatric medicine where great age is usually a contra-indication to meddlesome postponement of death by means of respirators, artificial kidneys and other techniques. Although active euthanasia is repugnant to many, dysthanasia* is usually avoidable whether due to natural causes or iatrogenic. As Card says, an individual might well describe the life of a member of his own family as priceless, whereas society often has to allot a monetary value to human life. However, an individual is often unselfish enough to value his or her own life, health, and comfort lower than a close relative's, a point worth considering when difficult choices have to be made; the individual's own attitude to euthanasia should be considered.

Brocklehurst, and Brotherston and Thom confidently predict a rise in the numbers and proportion of the elderly in the British population in the next 25 years. The very old make some of the heaviest demands on the National Health Service. This serious problem demands immediate medical, political and economic attention: it seems inevitable that the demands of the elderly will absorb increasing resources, which are likely to be diverted from elsewhere. Politics combined with community medicine could often be more of an experimental science than it usually is, and carefully devised and monitored pilot experiments might be done in a few randomly chosen areas of the country to evaluate possible ways of satisfying efficiently the needs of the elderly.

Queuing is one means of achieving rationing. It can operate in the context of a limited scarcity and strong community self-discipline. Appointments systems may result in long waiting times for a medical consultation and the traditional waiting list for admission or operation may be unrealistically long. Queuing could be reduced if resources were

*By dysthanasia, we mean dying with difficulty, unpleasantly or in pain.

concentrated more on easy efficient treatments and operations than on the more complicated and expensive in which benefit may be slight; this is an application of an economic theorem stated more generally below. Even the hotel function of a hospital is rarely required for investigations, but if so, pre-programming economizes on expensive beds (Brocklehurst). A small rise in the threshold of indications for observation, investigation, x-rays and relatively minor or marginally advisable treatment or operation would probably be ethically acceptable. It would allow some mitigation of the 'first come first served' method which has to be adopted even in some serious conditions such as renal failure.

Research is likely to be penalized disproportionately when resources become scarce, because research, especially laboratory research (Pickford), is so expensive and its results so unpredictable. The mobility of research workers allows them to go to countries where finance is more plentiful, to the possible detriment of their homelands. Originality is *the* quality to be selectively encouraged even in stringent times. However, an increased awareness of social relevance, for example by Black's 'indices of burden', and a more critical assessment of scientific feasibility may help to achieve greater effectiveness in this field. One of the main theorems of economics has an application to the dilemma which is discernible in these two chapters. When several choices are available, and maximization of returns, subject to constraints, is the aim, then priority should be given to those choices which will yield the greatest returns (given a fixed expenditure) rather than to those choices which would yield the greatest benefit if unlimited resources were applied to them. Various assumptions about externalities and distribution are implicit in that statement, but the basic principle should be clear.

Pickford lists in order of importance for research, diseases of circulation, brain and peripheral nervous systems, joints and muscles and skin. Some saving can be achieved by avoiding repetition and she points out the dangers of ignoring the literature of more than 25 years previously. At national level, some direction has always existed; but there should be enough inter-regional co-operation to avoid duplication, and to encourage more multicentre investigations. Some supranational co-ordination, at least with Europe and North America, should be possible. The expense of modern research equipment and its maintenance suggests inter-laboratory sharing as a means of achieving economies.

Conclusions

We would summarize a basis for long-term economies in clinical practice in these 10 points, which are applications of the Rule of Parsimony which we think should be applied in clinical management.

1. Each clinician must consider the total social cost of every resource which he employs, including apparently trivial items which can summate into large expenditures.

2. Medical undergraduates and established clinicians must be well informed about the cost of investigations and treatment.

3. Doctors should have more training in logic and statistics, particularly the basic common-sense principles of the randomized controlled clinical trial, and should be critical of routines.

4. Diseases which can be efficiently treated should attract much more resources than those in which benefit is slight and cost high.

5. Understaffing is an important and necessary principle for economy in medicine.

6. The general practitioner could accept more responsibility in the management of patients, and patients could reduce their own demands on the general practitioner.

7. Paramedical and lay personnel should replace the doctor where appropriate.

8. Surplus trainee posts should be eliminated; i.e. only enough general practitioners and specialists should be trained in the National Health Service to fill the anticipated number of permanent posts in it.

9. The increasing problem of geriatric care requires urgent solution, with pilot social experiments.

10. Dysthanasia* should be avoided. The subjective cut-off point should be decided by each clinician for his individual patient, particularly in relation to the patient's age and wishes.

We have attempted to make a case for critical selectivity and discriminating parsimony in the clinical management of patients. The resources saved could be employed elsewhere, not necessarily within the Health Service. This policy is logically and ethically attractive. It is a political necessity and an economic imperative.

*By dysthanasia, we mean dying with difficulty, unpleasantly or in pain.

Acknowledgements

Chapter 10. This chapter was written while the author was a Josiah Macy Jr Faculty Scholar, 1975-1976, at the Royal Postgraduate Medical School, London. It is based upon a McArthur Lecture given at the University of Edinburgh in June, 1976, and as part of a Festschrift in honour of Dr Richard L. Riley at Johns Hopkins Medical School in May, 1977. The author is grateful to Professor J.G. Scadding for his criticism of the manuscript.

Chapter 12. The author acknowledges with gratitude a supporting grant from the Scottish Home and Health Department.

Chapter 14. The author is indebted to many colleagues who have read this chapter and given advice, especially Dr Linda Beeley, Lecturer in Therapeutics and Clinical Pharmacology in his Department. He is also indebted to Mrs Maureen Roberts, Department of Statistics and Research, Department of Health and Social Security, for help with the Tables.

Chapter 18. The following are owed deep gratitude for advice and help willingly given: Dr E.H.I. Harries, Sir George Pickering FRS, Professor David Smyth FRS, Dr Andrew Swan, Dr D.E.M. Taylor, Dr A. Ungar, Dr P. Williams, Dr Alma B. Simmonds, Professor E.M. Symonds, Dr A. Hutton Wilson and Sir Gordon Wolstenholme FRS.

INDEX

The page containing most information is set in **heavy type**.